Making Babies the Hard Way

Living with Infertility and Treatment

Caroline Gallup

Foreword by William L. Ledger

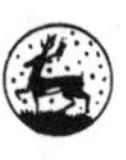

Jessica Kingsley Publishers
London and Philadelphia

'A Blade of Grass' on pp.96–7 from *Love Poems* (1991) by Brian Patten reprinted by permission of HarperCollins Publishers Ltd. © Brian Patten 1991
Quotation on p.97 from *The Writings of Nichiren Daishonin* (volume 1) (1999) published by Soka Gakkai reprinted by permission of Soka Gakkai. © Soka Gakkai 1999
Quotation on p.97 from *A Piece of Mirror and Other Essays* (2004) by Daisaku Ikeda reprinted by permission of Soka Gakkai. © Soka Gakkai 2004
Quotation on p.188 from *Conquering Infertility* (2002) by Alice D. Domar PhD and A. Lesch Kelly reprinted by permission.
The definitions in the Glossary from the *HFEA Guide to Infertility* (2006/2007) are reprinted by permission of HFEA.
The definitions in the Glossary from *Art of Living* are reprinted by permission of SGI-UK.

First published in 2007
by Jessica Kingsley Publishers
116 Pentonville Road
London N1 9JB, UK
and
400 Market Street, Suite 400
Philadelphia, PA 19106, USA

www.jkp.com

Library of Congress Cataloging in Publication Data
A CIP catalog record for this book is available from the Library of Congress

British Library Cataloguing in Publication Data
A CIP catalogue record for this book is available from the British Library

ISBN 978 1 84310 463 6

Printed and bound in Great Britain by
Athenaeum Press, Gateshead, Tyne and Wear

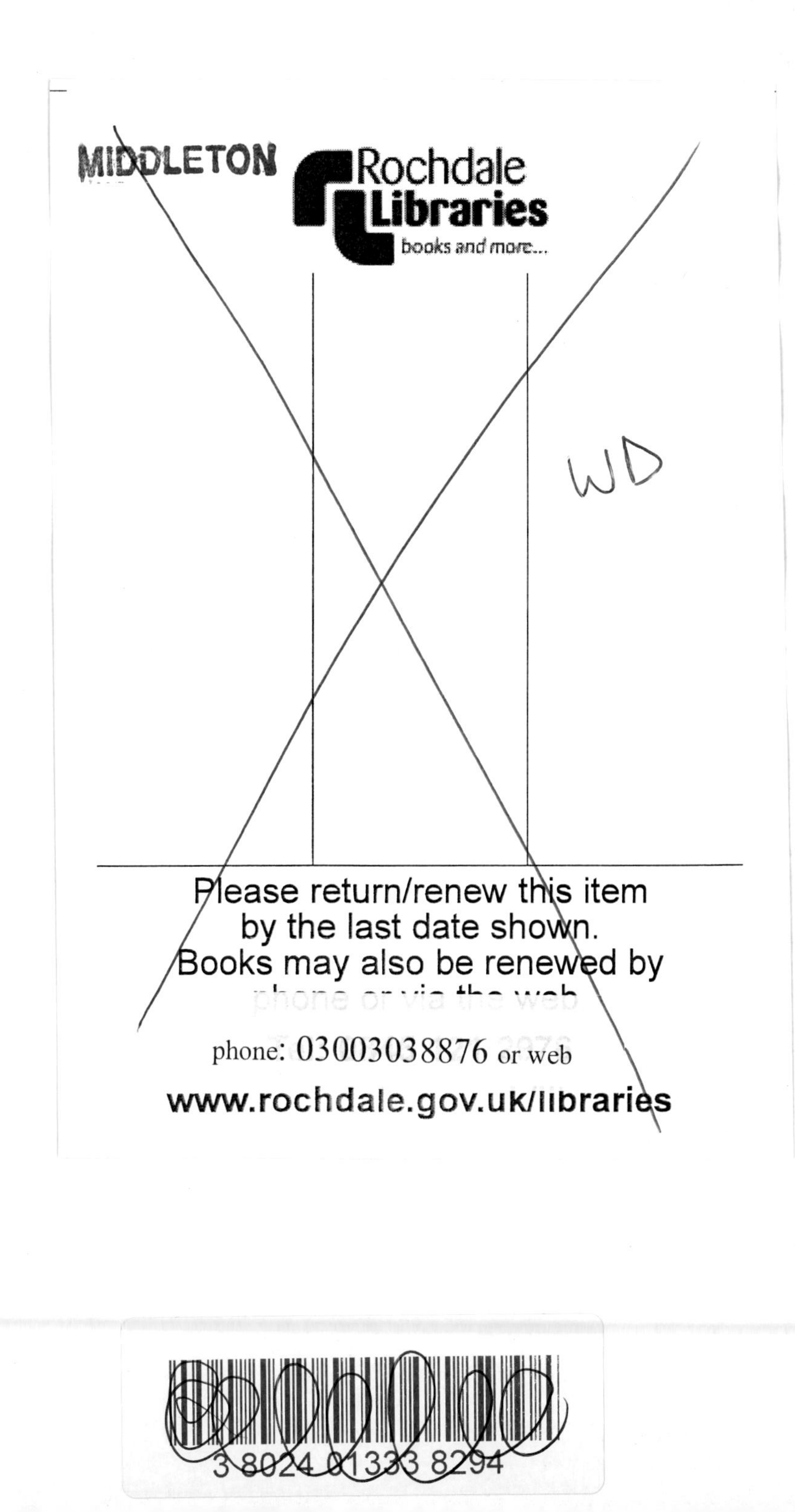

of related interest

Grief Unseen
Healing Pregnancy Loss through the Arts
Laura Seftel
Foreword by Sherokee Ilse
ISBN 978 1 84310 805 4

Sexuality and Fertility Issues in Ill Health and Disability
From Early Adolescence to Adulthood
Edited by Rachel Balen and Marilyn Crawshaw
ISBN 978 1 84310 339 4

Third Party Assisted Conception Across Cultures
Social, Legal and Ethical Perspectives
Edited by Eric Blyth and Ruth Landau
ISBN 978 1 84310 084 3 pb
ISBN 978 1 84310 085 0 hb

Experiences of Donor Conception
Parents, Offspring and Donors through the Years
Caroline Lorbach
Foreword by Eric Blyth
ISBN 978 1 84310 122 2

Fostering Now
Messages from Research
Ian Sinclair
Foreword by Tom Jeffreys, Director General, Children, Families and Young People Directorate, DfES
ISBN 978 1 84310 362 2

Relative Grief
Parents and Children, Sisters and Brothers, Husbands, Wives and Partners, Grandparents and Grandchildren Talk about their Experience of Death and Grieving
Clare Jenkins and Judy Merry
Foreword by Dorothy Rowe
ISBN 978 1 84310 257 1

For Bruce
One love – it's now!

Contents

Acknowledgements

My gratitude goes to many individuals and organizations that supported me during the writing of this book. Without them, this resource would not exist.

Thanks to Marianne Jones for being there for me for 36 years and counting – ours is an extraordinary friendship. Thanks and Canadian bear hugs for Heather Davies – your unfaltering daily support and insights nursed me through the hard times; onwards and upwards my friend. To Caroline Natzler, Renée Tyack and Barbara Rennie, whose invaluable input helped organize my hormonal ramblings – thanks for listening to draft, after draft, after draft, after draft. Thank you also to the City Lit autobiographical writing class of 2003/04, and to fellow writers in Caroline's smaller groups for pointing out the sections of my diaries worth developing.

My eternal gratitude goes to my mentor, Daisaku Ikeda, President of the Soka Gakkai, and to my wise and supportive family in faith – fellow SGI-UK members, particularly Sanda McWilliam, Sue Thornton, Sachiyo Wilson, Akemi Baynes, Jo Lane, Viv Moore, Cali Bird, Peter Osborn, Gayle Coleman, Kazuo Fujii and Robert Samuels, who at different times, in many different ways, have reminded me that it is always darkest just before the dawn, and that perseverance and being true to myself is bound to bring benefit.

To my fertility friends – they know who they are, but with special thanks to Paula, Susannah, Pauline, Kate, Yvonne and Nicky for listening and telling me of their own private struggles – you made me realize that I wasn't alone. I am also grateful to the numerous and equally valued dog owners and neighbours of our close-knit Brent community, who have been so supportive and compassionate during this time.

Thanks to everyone at the Bridge Centre, the London Fertility Centre, the Human Fertilisation and Embryology Authority (HFEA) and Infertility Network UK (I N UK), especially Pip Reilly, Dr Alan Thornhill, Ema Locker, Norah Harding, John Paul Maytum, Gosia Heeley and Andrew Berkeley, for their knowledge, vision and encouragement.

Thanks to the editors who gave me the breaks in my fledgling career, particularly Michele Lamb, whose compassion and training helped me to find my voice. Thanks to Stephen Jones, my editor at Jessica Kingsley Publishers, and my agent Tony Morris for your belief in this book, and your honesty and encouragement during the past two years. My thanks also go to the rest of the team at Jessica Kingsley, and to Jane Smith, for their fastidious attention to detail.

Thanks to HarperCollins and Brian Patten for their kind permission to publish 'A Blade of Grass', a poem that means a great deal to us. I am also grateful to Olivia and Walter Merricks, founders of the Donor Conception Network, whose series 'Planning a Family' was instrumental in increasing our understanding of the complexities and implications of using donor gametes. Information about their website and other useful addresses are printed at the back of this book.

I'd like to express my deepest gratitude to our friends and families who permitted their inclusion in this book – the story we wanted to tell would not have been possible without your generous and courageous agreement. Thanks also to Barney and Guz, my doggy pals who forced me to get out of bed and into the park on mornings when I would rather have pulled the duvet over my head.

Finally, to my husband, Bruce – your courage astounds me. Your contribution and support have been unwavering and unique. I love you for all eternity.

Foreword

This is a remarkable book. It describes one couple's journey along the rollercoaster pathway of treatment for infertility. What makes it different is the author's insight into her condition and her honest and perceptive descriptions of the impact of infertility on her and her partner. Caroline and Bruce find that their lack of fertility is due to 'male factor' – Bruce has no sperm. This is one of the most common yet least discussed causes of infertility, and Caroline's narrative is beautifully interrupted from time to time by Bruce's perspective on their treatment and its effects on them both. They describe a happy, stable relationship as a 'family of three' with Barney the dog, before the decision to try for a baby changes their lives. What follows is their experience of the various investigations, treatments and disappointments that comprise the modern management of infertility. The book is clearly written, and medical terms are carefully explained without disturbing the flow of the story.

I read this as a book about coping with infertility and its many consequences. Caroline and Bruce cope with the insensitivity and lack of knowledge of their GP, with adopting the 'patient' mindset (involving long waits to see doctors and nurses) and accepting intimate examinations and discussion of matters usually kept between partners; they cope with the physical pain of surgery and the emotional pain of repeated cycles of treatment that do not result in pregnancy. Caroline copes with her friends' pregnancies and children, their well-meaning but sometimes hapless attempts to sympathise with her infertility, and with people's assumption that it's 'her fault'. Above all, Caroline and Bruce eventually 'cope' with not having a family, the process of moving through treatment and reaching a point of closure of that part of their lives.

Caroline and Bruce take time to explore the impact of the various chapters of their infertility treatment on their lives and their relationship, from the graphic description of Bruce's testicular biopsies to the agonising over whether to accept treatment with donor insemination. This is a common dilemma and any couple faced with this choice would do well to learn from this text. The highs and lows of donor insemination treatment, monitoring of follicle growth and ovulation, and Caroline's exploration of and frustration with this aspect of her body's function will strike a chord with any woman who has followed this pathway. Caroline's list of things not to say to an infertile couple (and what helps) should be required reading for anyone who has experienced a 'foot in mouth' moment when struggling for the right words with a friend or colleague, and her advice to fellow-sufferers about how to communicate their infertility to family and friends is both practical and perceptive.

In the midst of this painful journey, Caroline and Bruce decide to marry, and the positivity and also the normality of this process contrasts with the medicalised world of the fertility clinic. Caroline's ability to paint such pictures brings the reader into her and Bruce's lives, and we feel their suffering as yet more treatments end in failure as further costly and complicated treatment does not produce the desired result. Caroline's self-knowledge allows her to explore the complicated emotional pressures that surface at times of life-altering decisions. I was pleased to read her largely positive description of her supportive counselling, along with her pithy observations (absolutely true) of the ubiquity of the potted palm and comfy chairs in the counselling environment. I was also impressed by her observations on the help she gained from websites run by the Human Fertility and Embryology Authority and various patient support groups. The Internet is often accused of doing more harm than good, but she shows how intelligent use of it can help patients understand more and cope better with their problem.

Caroline beautifully describes the reason that drives so many couples on through fertility treatment:

"The desire to have children is complex and so deeply ingrained in our biology that no one fully understands it until they meet a barrier to that desire."

I see this fundamental drive at work on a daily basis, its consequences for the couples involved and to their families. Infertility is incredibly common, yet still poorly understood. I would recommend this book to anyone who is facing infertility, or whose life has been touched by it. I will recommend it to my colleagues and students who see infertile couples as patients. If only this book could be read and understood by the fortunate fertile, there would be more compassion and understanding towards the infertile.

As Caroline and Bruce say: "If you approach a subject such as infertility with absolute openness, honesty and candour, you will be amazed by the reactions."

This is what she and her husband have done in this book. It will bring solace to many and understanding to many more.

Professor William L Ledger
Academic Unit of Reproductive and Developmental Medicine
University of Sheffield
March 2007

Introduction

The human capacity to love is the greatest force for good on Earth, and the love of a parent for their child one of the most universally recognized expressions of unconditional love across all cultures. To be denied this possibility is devastating, and a huge obstacle to overcome. This is true whether the denial is through the loss of a child, a miscarriage, termination or the inability to conceive in the first place. As nearly one in three of us know someone experiencing infertility or sub-fertility, it is crucially important to understand what it feels like and how to support someone going through it, whether that person is a loved one, friend, colleague or patient.

This book is a personal journey through fertility treatment and out the other side. It illustrates how the process may impact on daily life and relationships, whether you are a man or a woman. A large number of couples separate as a result of the strain placed on them by fertility treatment, even if the treatment has been successful. I hope that this book will help highlight how the stresses and strains may manifest – forewarned is forearmed.

Bruce and I had been together for six years when we decided the time was right for us to start a family. I was 38 years old; Bruce was 33. We were living in a one-bedroom garden flat, together with our dog Barney. Adopting Barney from Battersea Dogs' Home the previous year was the first step in our transition from being a couple to becoming a family. The interviewer approving us to be dog owners had written on our application form, 'These two will make wonderful parents.'

We hadn't been thoughtless in delaying the decision to have children; on the contrary, we felt that it was irresponsible to bring a new life into the world before we had enough time to devote to raising a child, enough living space to accommodate a family, and financial stability.

By making the decision to start a family, we, like millions of others, were trying to fulfil a natural desire. However, this expectation is becoming increasingly unrealistic as more than one in seven couples is affected by infertility worldwide; 3.5 million people in the UK are currently seeking advice on this issue. There is an assumption that in the majority of cases female factors are to blame, but this is incorrect, as problems caused by male infertility are currently at the same level and, some believe, rising at a faster rate. This book will help you and those who know you to understand and cope with the challenges fertility treatment presents. It will encourage you to ask questions and to feel more confident about making the right choices for you.

Almost 80 per cent of couples undergoing assisted conception treatments currently remain unsuccessful, and have to face the agonizing decision of when and how to draw a line under the process. It may take many years to accept a future that is different from the one they had planned. We do not advocate any single solution, merely that the most important achievement is to make the right decision for you, whatever that may be.

The diaries on which this book is based were written over a four-year period, beginning mid-way through 2001. For clarity of themes and narrative, some names have been changed, characters merged and time condensed. Bruce has contributed his own viewpoint to the narrative, and where this occurs his voice appears in a different font.

My aim is to give you an insight into some of the rigours and excitement you will experience when opting for fertility treatment, and to show that you can be happy, whatever the outcome.

1

'It doesn't make you any less of a man you know'

We haven't had to wait long to see our doctor – just enough time to thumb through the mix of high-brow, low-brow and children's magazines on the table; to read all the government health campaign posters and to get uncomfortable on the cheap white-plastic chairs. The receptionist calls our names. As we enter the doctor's office, she is finishing off some paperwork. 'How can I help you today?' she asks, without looking up.

We sit down as she spins to face us in her swivel chair and smiles. I can see that Bruce is feeling awkward having to explain.

'We're here to get my sperm test results… Ahem…' He clears his throat, then averts his gaze slightly. 'We're trying to have a baby… I had a virus and had to repeat my last sperm test.'

'Righty-ho,' she exclaims, as she cheerfully swivels back to face the computer screen on her desk.

There is an anxious silence because the computer won't give up the information. After a few exasperated groans, she triumphs.

'Ah. There we are,' she says, peering into the monitor. She pauses before saying, 'There aren't any.'

'Aren't any what?' I'm confused – no records, no results, no *what?*

'No sperm I'm afraid.'

She's still wearing that smile; why is she smiling?

'What, none at all?' I feel my eyes pleading with the doctor for a different response. Bruce is looking at the floor. His face is flushed and he's not saying anything.

'Is this common?' I ask.

'No, not really,' she replies.

The doctor is looking at Bruce, who appears to have 'checked out' of the situation. I want to give his hand a squeeze, but I can't move.

'Is there anything we can do?'

'No, I don't think there is I'm afraid.' *At least she's stopped smiling.*

'Now I hate to jump the gun Caroline, but – donor sperm...'

What is she talking about? What about Bruce? I want to shout out: 'It's *his* baby I want.' How can she expect me to simply move on to using donor sperm, without investigation or explanation? Donor sperm – I can't do that. Why would I want to do that?

I watch Bruce re-cross his legs and shift his weight, sinking deeper into the chair. The doctor notices as well, because she turns to him and says, 'It doesn't make you any less of a man you know.'

I try to slow down my thoughts, regain some composure and take control of this situation.

'What might have caused this, doctor?'

'Well, we don't really know.'

'Isn't there *anything* we can do?'

'I'm sorry. I really don't think there is.'

The consultation seems to be coming to an end, but we stay sitting down, unable to move. We want something more from her. She *must* know more than this. I don't know what the questions are, but there must *be* some. The doctor rises out of her chair, walks across to the sink and begins washing her hands. I try for more information, for a way to deal with this body blow.

'Is there any counselling available to us?' I ask.

'Well, I suppose so, if you think you want it...'

'Is anyone carrying out research?' There may be some new advance that she isn't aware of yet – infertility seems to be on the television and in the newspapers virtually every week.

'Well there are one or two, but I don't think they've got very far.' She doesn't turn around.

Poor Caro, she's doing her best and asking every question she can think of, but the doctor is not being very helpful. I can hear their conversation continuing, but it's going on somewhere outside of me – I don't feel a part of it. *'Aren't any what?'* I'm fairly sure that if I could just get out into the cool evening air my face would feel normal again. All the blood in my body seems to be rushing to my cheekbones, and my eyes feel hot.

I just want to be out of here – *'Is this common?'* – on the top of the hill, in the park, kicking a ball for our dog Barney to chase. I can see him racing back towards me, his ears flapping, his tongue lolling out of the side of his mouth. 'Here boy, come here boy.'

I snap back into the room as I hear the words, 'It doesn't make you any less of a MAN you know.' I can't think of anything to say to this woman. This doesn't seem to have any meaning. If only I can just get out of here. I just want to be home.

The doctor finishes drying her hands, and comes to sit down again. 'Well, I think we'll have to leave it there,' she says.

I'm furious with our GP and worried about Bruce, but I hear myself saying 'Thank you' as we rise out of the seats and leave. But what am I thanking her for? What are we going to do?

The day we met

I found love, quite unexpectedly, at a run-of-the-mill business meeting. I was working as a theatre production manager. A friend of mine had written a musical and asked me to look after the technical and financial side of things whilst a mutual friend was to direct. Graham, the director, responded to our search for a set designer by inviting 'an exciting young designer called Bruce Gallup' to our meeting.

I walked into the room and THWACK! – the velvet boxing glove of love hit me. Meeting Bruce gave me an extraordinary feeling of coming home. I felt excited and light-headed – as if I was floating just above the floorboards. *So there you are then. I've been waiting for you.*

I drank in his soft green eyes, his long, fair, wavy hair, tied back in a ponytail; broad shoulders and that smile – to me, he was perfect. I squealed inside when he asked for my phone number at the end of the meeting. I didn't believe in love at first sight, but still I went home and waited for his call. I even told my friend Penny that I'd met 'The One'.

The phone didn't ring in December. It didn't ring in the January, or February. I assumed that I must have been mistaken about his feelings for me, but then, one evening in March, halfway through a girls' night-in with Penny, the phone rang.

'Hello, it's Bruce. I don't know whether you remember me, but a gang of us are driving over to France for the weekend. Would you like to join us?'

'It's *him*,' I mimed, theatrically pointing to the handset. Penny clapped her hands together in excitement.

I feigned affront. 'Don't you think you're being a bit cheeky after all this time?'

'Well, I just thought I'd ask. It might be fun.' He didn't seem discouraged.

'Oh, okay then, since you put it so nicely.' I tried to sound cool.

One week later, we headed off in convoy to Dover for the crossing to France. Bruce drove his dark-green, open-topped sports car and bought me chocolates and flowers. Could it get any better than this?

My life changed when I met Caroline. I wasn't looking for a long-term relationship; I was living in the same, shared flat above an opticians in South London that I had moved into after leaving art school six years before. Most of my time was committed to work, but any fleeting liaison that might occur as a by-product was okay by me. It wasn't that I didn't want to share my life in the long term, but there didn't seem to be room for anyone and I couldn't imagine it being possible. I guess I was pretty self-absorbed.

Why things changed I don't really know. Maybe it was the combination of the right time and the right person. I still don't know to this day why I asked Caro to come to France with me. There was no real plan, except that I thought she seemed like fun. I wanted to be in her company.

We landed in Calais, ate *croque-monsieur*, drank cheap champagne and I inflicted my schoolgirl French on the long-suffering locals.

In the sunshine on the beach at Le Touquet, he taught me how to fly kites. As we watched the sun go down, I smiled inwardly at our unexpected meeting and looked forward to a relationship with Bruce in which anything was possible.

By the time we'd bought our first place together and began trying for a baby, we felt that we already knew our child. The decision to get pregnant was preceded by occasional light-hearted fantasies about how a child with a mix of our genes would look. Of course he or she would be *devastatingly* attractive, we joked between ourselves. We imagined our child having fair curly hair and blue or green eyes. He or she might be artistic, sporty, musical or have an aptitude for science – all of these traits feature on both sides of our families. The only feature proving a challenge to imagine was our child's nose, as mine is bordering on the retroussé, whilst Bruce's is a more prominently sculpted family attribute.

Imagining what having a child would be like, I checked out nursery schools and we talked excitedly about tobogganing on trays down the hill in the nearby park and taking 'junior' to the kid's football club we saw as we walked Barney there on Saturdays. Bruce planned to pass on his love of rugby whether our children were boys or girls; I would be responsible for nature trips and holidays.

My vision of our child was further strengthened because of my faith. I am a Buddhist; a member of an organization known as Soka Gakkai International (SGI) and have been chanting and studying the teachings of a Japanese priest named Nichiren Daishonin since 1995. Bruce is not Buddhist, but wholeheartedly supports my practice as he can see the benefit I gain from this philosophy. Over the years, through chanting, I have become used to developing clarity of thought or insight into what I want for my life or seeing the steps I need to take to overcome whatever problem is challenging me. I find it a practical approach to problem solving. But on one occasion I had an extraordinary experience.

I had been chanting strongly for about 20 minutes or so in the main hall at one of our European centres when I sensed a toddler standing beside me. Of course, I knew that no child was physically there, and yet, I could 'see' a blond, curly-haired boy of around three years old. He smiled at me, then crouched down and turned slightly away, as if he wanted me to get out of my seat and chase after him. 'Come on, Mum! Hurry up, it'll be fun!' He ran mischievously between the rows of chairs, zigzagging in and out of the aisles, full of energy. He was delightful. I continued to chant for another five minutes or so, enjoying the sense of this energetic toddler inhabiting my thoughts. When I stopped chanting I was smiling, inside and out. I interpreted this 'vision' as a sign that our time to be parents was imminent and inevitable. I had met our future son.

During the following year back at home in North West London, we used our hard-won financial stability to stretch ourselves . We put in an offer on a four-bedroom family house a few streets away from our one-bed garden flat. I resigned my demanding job as an event manager at the Royal Albert Hall to set up my own event services company, working from home. Bruce made a career move out of theatre design and into the more challenging, but lucrative, film industry as a special effects and scenic painter. We calculated that by the time our baby came along, my business would be established, enabling me to work more flexible hours and perhaps afford to bring in staff for extra help. Bruce was potentially capable of making up any temporary shortfall in our joint income whilst I was coping with being a new mum.

We were both aware that being 38 years old, with a history of erratic ovulation and treatment seven years ago for abnormal cervical cells, meant that getting pregnant might take some time. Mr Parkes, the gynaecologist who had removed the pre-cancerous cells and monitored me until the previous year, always made sure I knew the facts.

'After the age of 38, fertility falls by half in women,' he warned. 'If you don't get pregnant within six months, ask your GP to run some fertility tests. Usually couples are asked to try for one year before seeking advice, but with your history you should try to get help sooner rather than later.'

I've had no recurrence of suspect cells since the operation and my ovulation has settled down to a regular pattern, so I no longer see Mr Parkes on a regular basis, but I have always remembered his advice.

After six months of trying, but no pregnancy, we made an appointment with the local surgery, but were not able to see our own GP. The locum took blood from me to test hormone levels and, much to his embarrassment, Bruce had to take a semen sample to our local hospital so that it could be tested for volume and motility of sperm.

The results of my first batch of tests – carried out in September – surprised us by being normal. My levels of follicle-stimulating hormone (FSH) were below ten, which is a good indicator of fertility (notwithstanding blocked tubes or other problems). But Bruce's first sperm test results were mystifying – there were no sperm present in the sample he had provided. The locum, who told us she had a special interest in this area of medicine, dismissed our concerns by saying that this was not unusual. Referring to Bruce's notes, she told us that the virus he had recently contracted could have killed all the sperm: 'Sperm take three months to "re-stock". Wait until the New Year and then do another test. I'll give you a sample bottle today and we'll send the result to your home.'

With that, we left her office and waited to test again. October, November, December – still my monthly periods showed that I wasn't pregnant. Disappointing as this was, we remembered the doctor's reassurances, so when January arrived, Bruce made yet another dash to the local hospital, keeping the sperm warm by transporting the sample bottle under his armpit as he'd been told to do.

Ten days later, an envelope post-marked from our surgery dropped onto the doormat. Inside was an automated computer print out, which started 'Dear [Blank]'. It then offered some options, most of which I have forgotten, but I do remember words to the effect of: (a) make an appointment to see the GP to discuss this further, (b) repeat test, (c) go away and stop making such a fuss, there's nothing wrong with you.

I remember the 'Repeat test' option vividly, because it was absent-mindedly circled, the black biro barely encompassing the two words. It ended impersonally with a rubber stamp.

'What's *this* supposed to mean?' Bruce asked, waggling the paper for me to see. 'You'd think they'd have taken more trouble. What was the result of the test? Do I have to see them again before I do a third test or what?'

'Look, don't worry,' I said. 'Just do the test. I'll go and collect another sample bottle from the surgery this afternoon. At the same time, I'll make an appointment with our regular GP. I'm sure she will be able to give us more information.'

★ ★ ★

Bruce hasn't spoken since we received the third test result. We drive the short distance back to our flat in silence. I don't want to push him to say anything, in case he just wants to be quiet – he must be devastated.

As we open the front door to the house and the internal door into our apartment, Barney pushes his nose through to greet us. Wagging his tail enthusiastically, he turns and leads us down the hallway, into our box-filled sitting room – it's ironic that we're moving to our new family house soon. Bruce lights the fire, I open a bottle of red wine and we sit on the floor, either side of the fireplace, looking blankly at each other.

I break the silence, but as the words tumble out, I'm shocked at the strength of my feelings.

'I'm sorry, but I can't do donor sperm. I find the idea repulsive. I've been trying to imagine what it would feel like. First someone else's sperm...and then someone else's child growing in *my* body...ugh... Like something left over after... I know this sounds extreme, but I think I'd feel as if something sordid had happened to me. I feel ashamed for thinking that, but I just can't do it.'

What an awful thing to say. As soon as I've spoken, I regret what I've said. Poor Bruce. I should have been more positive – or sensitive.

'Sorry,' I say, looking down at the floor. I'm really struggling with the doctor's pronouncement. Because of my vision, I had convinced myself that we would definitely have our own child one day. Given what we know now, evidently that little boy was just a ridiculous fantasy.

Bruce is poking the flames with a fire-iron. He has always said that hearths and home fires tend to bring back happy memories of childhood trips with his father, collecting logs in their old mini-van. His dad wore a holey old jumper reserved specifically for doing 'just jobs' around the house and in the garage. Father and son would do DIY together: they have rebuilt garden walls, sorted out the vegetable patch and worked on various clapped-out old jalopies bought by Bruce with his teenage savings.

When Bruce finally speaks, his thoughts are just as primitive as my own: 'The Gallup line will end with me then.' Bruce has two sisters and four female cousins.

I don't know what else to say. All our fantasies about how a child with the combination of our genes might look have evaporated. No family resemblance. No more guessing to look forward to. There is a vast chasm between us and we are both staring into the void.

Discovering options

Still only halfway through my glass of wine and staying warm by the fire, I try to find ways to accept the situation. 'Perhaps we'd feel better if the sperm donor wasn't anonymous?' I suggest.

We desperately search through Bruce's relatives for someone to ask. There is a male relative on his mother's side, but we hardly know him. We try to think of anyone else, but realize that Bruce's father is the only other candidate – and recoil from this idea, as the child would be Bruce's brother. 'Anyway, can you imagine how embarrassing it would be asking him?' We recoil in horror at the thought. Whilst Bruce re-fills our glasses, I have another idea: 'I'm going to give Mr Parkes a call. He might be able to suggest something.'

Although he had never met Bruce, Mr Parkes always said to phone him with any problems if I thought he could help. I figure that he must know something, or some*one*, who can help us.

I dial his number, and wait for him to pick up. He is surprised to hear from me at this late hour. 'Hello Mr Parkes. I hope that you won't mind me calling, but I really need some advice...'

I explain our situation and apparent lack of options.

'Oh dear, I'm so sorry about your results, but it's not an absolute dead-end. There are things you can do.'

After 20 minutes of note scribbling and absorbing his recommendations, I put the phone down and turn back to Bruce.

'Basically, the first thing we need to do is to get you to see a urologist or an andrologist.' I scan my notes to find the information. 'They're specialists in the male reproductive system, and male infertility. You could have a blockage preventing sperm getting out, which they might be able to clear. They can also take tissue samples from where the sperm are made, and if they find any, they can use them to fertilize one of my eggs. Apparently they only need one sperm. They'd inject it directly into my egg. It's called – hang on, it's here somewhere – intra-cytoplasmic sperm injection – ICSI for short. It's a relatively new technique, but Mr Parkes says they are getting good results.'

Bruce is still listening whilst sipping his wine. I take his relaxed mood as permission to continue.

'Mr Parkes also recommends that we go back to the GP and ask for a referral. I need to check the NHS [National Health Service] waiting list with the hospital once we have a name. If it's 13 weeks or more, it's worth paying to see someone privately so that we can speed things along. Otherwise, by the time they know what's wrong, I could be too old for treatment. I may even be too old already. Honestly, why didn't our GP tell us about these options?'

'Maybe she didn't know,' allows Bruce. 'But you're right, we have to do something, we mustn't be defeated – that's just not us.'

Bruce puts his glass down on the table, stands and walks over into our open-plan kitchen. 'Let's look on the bright side sweetheart. The GP may have pulled the rug out from under us, but hey, we've discovered there are floorboards underneath.'

2

'When will I be a grandma?'

The urology consultant

Mr Parkes' concerns about appointment waiting times were justified. For Bruce to see a urologist on the NHS would have taken 13 weeks. What's more, thanks to the lack of knowledge at our local surgery, when I rang to make a private appointment to speed things up, I found that we had been referred to the wrong specialist. Had I not been so impatient, we would have been waiting for more than three months to see a consultant who didn't specialize in male infertility. Thankfully the 'wrong' consultant gave me the name of the man we are about to see right now.

We're sitting in the third-floor waiting room of a vast private hospital in London's Harley Street. The room resembles the annexe to a hunting lodge: deep red carpet, tartan-covered wingback chairs, and a mahogany umbrella stand in the corner. I'm wondering how Bruce is feeling, but decide not to ask. He looks unflustered as usual, reading an issue of *Country Life* magazine. I hope it's not a farming article on artificial insemination. I'm feeling good – grateful to be getting somewhere, hopeful that there has been some kind of mistake about the sperm tests, or that something can be done for Bruce.

Bruce's name is called, so we walk together into the consulting room. The consultant extends his hand towards us across the mahogany desk: 'Hello. I'm Mr Liddiard. Please take a seat,' he smiles.

We explain the results of the tests so far. The specialist suggests that Bruce provides a fourth sperm sample and a blood test today, in the hospital.

'This will eliminate any possibility that the previous tests were somehow damaged in transit between home and your local hospital,' he says. 'The blood test will establish hormone levels; the levels of the follicle-stimulating hormone in men can give an indication of sperm production levels.'

The urologist ushers Bruce into an examination room off to one side of the office. I hear a curtain being drawn and various instructions being given during the examination. Bruce coughs loudly once or twice and they return to the main office after about ten minutes.

'Not the largest testicles I've ever seen,' says the urologist as they sit back down. *Well I bet that makes Bruce feel good. Thanks a bunch, Mr Liddiard.*

He goes on to explain that the size of testicles combined with high levels of FSH could mean that Bruce has *never* produced sperm. He needs to carry out more tests, but Bruce is already leaping ahead to a possible solution.

'Can you artificially manipulate the hormone levels maybe, to stimulate sperm production?'

'It doesn't work like that, unfortunately. FSH and sperm production aren't connected in that way. The levels are only an indicator of what *may* be going on in the body. Manipulating one doesn't affect the performance of the other – it's merely a by-product, in the same way that carbon dioxide is a by-product of breathing.'

That's it then. We're scuppered aren't we?

The specialist continues: 'There is an investigation you can have, which I would recommend. There's still a slim chance that all doors aren't shut. Once we've seen your results, we can discuss your options in more detail.'

He gives us the paperwork for the tests before stepping out from behind his desk to open the office door for us. We thank him for his time and take the elevator downstairs. Bruce takes my hand as the doors slide open, bringing us outside the laboratory.

'I do feel we're getting somewhere now,' he says. 'Actually, I feel quite positive. After seeing the GP, I felt useless. At least with this man we have information, and I don't feel like the only person in the world that this has happened to. The worst part was having my prostate checked – I could have done without that little surprise.'

Mum arrives

With great timing, not only are we completing on the purchase of our house today, but we also have to sneak out to see Mr Liddiard in Harley Street to get the results of Bruce's tests. Because of the house move over the next couple of days, we're soon to be surrounded by people wanting to help, namely Bruce's friend Ian, my best friend Marianne and my mum, who arrives this afternoon.

I can't face telling Mum about this yet; I'm still trying to absorb it myself. We may even be jumping to mistaken conclusions: there won't be anything to tell her if Bruce has a blockage rather than a complete absence of sperm. There's no sense in making a fuss over nothing.

The doorbell rings, heralding my mother's arrival. Barney wakes up with a start and runs down the hallway, barking.

'Good boy, that's enough now.' I shout for the dog to be quiet.

I open the door and give Mum a kiss on the cheek. She beams her smile at me, squinting slightly as she doesn't choose to wear her glasses all the time – 'Sometimes darling, life looks better through a haze.'

My mother, Betty, is a powerhouse of love – five feet two inches of energy, surrounded by a personality, face and figure belying her seventy-something years of age. She's been the champion of my life, a brilliant mum, but I've always felt sad about the hand that she was dealt in other ways. She never knew her elder sister, who died, from meningitis, before Mum was born. Her own mother died of pneumonia when infant Betty was only five months old. Her own father had to move away from Yorkshire to the south of England to find work. He wanted to send for her, but the Second World War kept them apart. Despite this separation, she had a happy childhood, raised by her grandmother, along with cousins, uncles and aunts, in a boisterous, laughter-filled home.

Mum loves children and they love her. She wanted two or three children of her own – armfuls of children to love – but this was prevented by my father's decision to change career and become a doctor when they were already eight years into their marriage. Sacrifices had to be made, so I'm an only child. My father passed away more than ten years ago; Mum is now retired.

I have always wanted to fill her life with grandchildren, to make amends somehow for her unfulfilled dreams. So I'm dreading telling her that she may never be 'grandma'. It's harder still because she is so thrilled for us about the house; we've finally got the space to start a family.

Teas in hand, we sit together on the sofa.

'How are you then sweetheart? All packed I see,' she comments wryly, as she surveys the blatant disorganization. Too confused and uncomfortable about fibbing to her to want much of a conversation, I mumble something about being busy with work, being glad of her help, gulp down my tea, get up and dive into my office. It won't be long now before Bruce comes home and we have to leave for Harley Street.

Later that day

It's BAD news; the worst news possible. Bruce's fourth sperm test confirms a total lack of sperm, *plus* a high level of FSH in his blood. I don't know what I'd hoped for, but each time we've been told, it's as if it's the first time I've heard it. Bruce must feel like he's been punched to the ground. His eyes are expressionless, but he's chewing his bottom lip, causing his jaw to clench and a ridge to appear in his cheek.

The consultant discreetly steps out of the room for a moment. I lean over to Bruce, taking hold of his hand between mine. 'How do you feel?'

He looks into my eyes. 'Not sure… It never really crossed my mind before… I suppose because of the build-up to today, I'm not surprised really… Mostly, I don't feel anything… I don't know what I feel.'

As Mr Liddiard comes back into the room, we both shift in our seats. I uncross my legs, placing my feet neatly and squarely on the floor, Bruce adjusts his jacket and smoothes a stray strand of his hair back into place.

'Have I always been like this?' he asks.

'Well, we don't know that you have a zero count for certain yet. You may be producing sperm; there could be an obstruction, which is usually correctable. But I have to warn you that in my experience hormone levels up in the twenties, combined with small testicles, usually points to a lack of sperm production. If this were caused by a blockage, we would expect to see FSH levels of ten or below.'

'What could have caused this?' Bruce asks.

Oh no, poor Bruce, he's started to blame himself. He can't possibly think this is somehow his fault can he?

'There could be a number of reasons, Mr Gallup. Part of your Y chromosome could be missing or damaged. There are various none-too-scientific theories about oestrogen in the water we drink, the possible effects of pesticides, chemicals in the soil, and so on, but there is no hard evidence to support…'

'I work with paints and solvents,' Bruce interrupts. 'There's supposed to be oestrogen in paint…and I don't always wear gloves. Is this something I could have prevented?'

Mr Liddiard explains that working with various chemicals and substances may contribute to a low sperm count, as does smoking and drinking alcohol, but to a *low* rather than a *no* sperm count. He urges us not to speculate, as there is no hard evidence to support any of those theories.

'So I haven't done anything to cause this?' asks Bruce.

'It's unlikely,' the consultant replies. 'It's best not to speculate in any event. Down that road…'

'Lies madness?' interrupts Bruce.

'Exactly. Thinking along those lines will only make you blame yourself when blame cannot necessarily be apportioned.'

We're told that the most likely cause in Bruce's case is that he has never produced sperm and has been this way since birth.

'For your own peace of mind,' Mr Liddiard continues, 'I suggest that you go onto the website of the Human Fertilisation and Embryology Authority – the HFEA. Have you heard of them? They're the licensing body monitoring all the clinics in the UK. Their website lists every licensed fertility centre. Go and see a specialist and ask for a testicular biopsy. Then you'll be able to see if any sperm exist in the testicle. If they do, they may be able to extract one to use in an ICSI, to fertilize one of Caroline's eggs.'

'How do we know which are the best clinics; the most successful?' I ask.

'The HFEA publish league tables for each of the procedures available. You can look up the figures for ICSI and IVF – you've heard of in-vitro fertilization?'

'That's fertilizing the egg and sperm outside the body isn't it?'

'That's right, hence the nickname "test tube baby". You should also look up donor insemination – DI. If Bruce doesn't have any sperm at all, you will need to use donor sperm. Get the percentage success rates in your age group, then contact the clinics with the greatest rates of success.'

Just before we descend onto the underground, I remember the situation at home.

'What about Mum? What are we going to tell her when we get back?'

'Well, she thinks that we've been to the solicitors to sign some papers for the house, so let's just say that it's all done, all fine, and keep all this to ourselves for now.'

'If that's what you want, that's fine by me honey.'

'Yes, I think so, for the moment. Don't you? If your mum and our friends weren't around right now, we'd probably choose to keep this to ourselves.'

'You're right,' I reply. 'Let's concentrate on moving and then think about what to do once we've looked at the HFEA website.'

Mum is oblivious to our subterfuge as we busy ourselves with the packing. When she offers to sleep overnight at the new house, with Barney for protection, we leap at the opportunity to have more time to ourselves.

Bruce runs Mum down the road, leaving me at the flat to go through the empty rooms and check for forgotten items. When he returns, I open a bottle of wine, attempting to celebrate our new purchase. But disappointment soon overwhelms me: 'There are four bedrooms in the new house. What on earth are we going to do with four bedrooms if we can't have children?'

We sit on the sofa close together, hold onto each other and cry.

★ ★ ★

Moving day, and Marianne, my best friend for over 30 years, has offered her services as chief box organizer. She walks past me in the hallway and goes into the sitting room, observing my red-rimmed eyes. 'Heavy night?' she asks.

'We didn't get much sleep.' I follow her through to the sitting room and kitchen.

Entering the sitting room, she looks aghast: 'Caroline, what a mess!'

There are empty boxes everywhere and the cupboard doors are open, still full of jars, tins and packets.

'I know, I know. We didn't get very far last night. We did do a lot of drinking and crying though. Look Marianne, I've got something to tell you. You'd better sit down. Quick, before my mum comes back here.'

I tell her about the tests and the prognosis and explain that I don't know what to do about Mum, as I can't face telling her yet. I don't want to have to think about how to break it to her, or her response.

Marianne looks shocked at first, then puts her arms around me.

'Oh mate, I'm so sorry. I'm not going to tell you everything is all right, because it's not, is it?'

I shake my head. 'I don't know how I'm going to cope with everything that needs to be done today. I feel absolutely wrecked.'

'You must be so sad.'

I step backwards, leaving her hand resting gently on my arm as I force the tears back behind my eyes and choke the lump away from my throat. She gives me a big hug, then looks around the room at the chaos, puts down her small rucksack, takes off her coat and hands it to me.

'Here you are. Hang this up somewhere it won't get packed, and go and make us a sandwich. I'll go into the bedroom and make a start on the clothes. When your mum gets here, send her to me – I'll keep her busy.'

What a relief. I keep my head down for the rest of the day, as I ferry Marianne back and forth to the new house with boxes. On the final trip, I realize that I don't want to keep hiding this from my mum any longer, so I ask Bruce if I can tell her tonight. He bravely agrees, suggesting that I engineer a final trip to the old flat to be alone with her.

Breaking the news

It's dark outside, and cold, but I feel flushed and my heart is thumping. I haven't really worked out what I'm going to say, but I have to do it. My mouth opens and I hear myself speaking.

'Mum, I have something to tell you.'

She's looking anxiously at me and I sense that she's anticipating bad news. I take a deep breath in, slowly breathe out and continue.

'You know that Bruce and I have been trying to have a baby?'

'Is anything wrong? Are you pregnant? Have you lost the baby? Oh, darling…'

Mum looks really concerned.

'No, no it's nothing like that,' I say, but I know she's not going to be reassured for long – it's only going to get worse.

'So, what is it?'

'Well, you see, we've been having tests to find out why I haven't become pregnant. It seems that Bruce could be infertile. If he is, we won't be able to have any children of our own at all.'

She looks sad, but corrects herself, looks me straight in the eye and says, 'Well, my love, it's not the end of the world you know. Children aren't everything.'

I start to cry again, partly from the relief of being honest with her.

'Oh my darling,' she says, as she puts her arms around me. 'Come on now, you've got Bruce; you're happy and you love each other. That's all that really matters.'

'But I know how much you wanted grandchildren; I wanted to give you grandchildren,' I sob into her shoulder.

'Oh, don't worry about me. I've got you and Bruce, and Barney. He's my furry grandson isn't he? I can make a fuss of *him* when I come to visit!'

I am so relieved. All the pressure I'd put on myself to be the perfect daughter is suddenly released. The first hurdle is over and I have unconditional love.

3

'You may feel a little uncomfortable for a few days'

Finding the right clinic

I've been doing some research of my own into male infertility. Bruce may never have produced sperm due to a microdeletion – a missing piece of his Y chromosome. In their book *Overcoming Male Infertility*, Leslie Schover and Anthony J. Thomas say that in up to 18 per cent of men who have no sperm at all, this piece of genetic information is either damaged or missing. No one knows why it happens; there are often no visible symptoms or indications of the condition and nothing can be done to correct it. But I'm not giving up hope. I've found the website recommended by the urologist, the Human Fertilisation and Embryology Authority – or the Hope For Everyone Association, as I like to call it.

I click first on *Information Sections, For Patients, Find a Clinic*, then *DI Clinics*. Go, little search engine.

Results found: 21 clinics specializing in DI and ICSI. Fantastic. Here are the league tables. The specialist advised us to try those that are successful in my age group. That, and the location, narrows it down a little.

The success rates don't actually seem so bad after the age of 38: IVF less than 30 per cent; ICSI, about the same. Not brilliant, but at least there's a chance.

I go back to the Home page, to see what else I can find out. 'For patients, find a clinic, type in your town or postcode, select a region, select a treatment type.' There are so many options: ICSI; DI; IVF; gamete intra-fallopian transfer (GIFT); storage of eggs; storage of sperm; storage of embryos; egg sharing; genetic screening.

The urologist said that we needed DI and ICSI, so I'll select those. Presumably I don't need to tick storage of eggs or sperm – I assume they'll have somewhere to put them if they carry out the other procedures! Oh well, I can always ask. No more to do for now; back to bed I think. I'll call the clinics first thing tomorrow morning.

★ ★ ★

It's only 9.30 a.m. I've been calling clinics since opening time half an hour ago, but I've had to break off and call Bruce. I'm so frustrated. He answers after only a couple of rings.

'Hello love, how are you doing?' he says.

'The clinics are driving me crazy already,' I reply. I tell Bruce how the first three I've spoken to insist that we are assessed together. They won't see him on his own. Last night, we agreed to confirm his diagnosis before we went any further, so that we would avoid repeating tests unnecessarily and wasting our limited funds. So far, all the clinics have told me that their policy is to investigate me as well.

'But that's silly. We may not want to proceed any further if my diagnosis is conclusive infertility.'

'I know. It just seems to me like another way to get money out of us. I've told them that I've already had all the blood tests, and that I'm okay, so why do I have to do them again? It's ridiculous. I have a couple more to try – I'll see what they have to say and ring you back.'

'Okay, lovely. Speak to you later. I love you.'

'I love you too. Call you later.'

I call the next clinic on my list – also the most straightforward in terms of travelling distance.

'Good morning, can I help you?'

'Yes, I hope so. We have been told that my partner is infertile, and have been advised by a consultant that there are more investigations available to us, to find out whether or not this is true. Can we make an appointment to see a specialist?'

'Yes of course. Our specialist in male infertility is called Mr Lambert. The next clinic is in two weeks' time. I can book your partner in if you like.'

'Thank you. That sounds great. His name's Mr Bruce Gallup. You don't need to see me at this stage?'

'No, that won't be necessary, although if you can accompany your partner, to provide the doctor with as full a picture as possible, that would be helpful. Mr Gallup will need two appointments, one for the consultation and one for an investigation. Is that okay?'

'Oh, yes of course. No problem.' *Poor Bruce – more prodding and poking.*

She clarifies our conversation. 'I'll make the appointments for Friday the fifth of next month, at four o'clock, and Saturday the sixth at 11. Is that okay?'

'That's fine, thank you. We'll see you in two weeks.'

Our first visit to a fertility clinic

The tube journey is short, and the directions easy to follow: out of the station, walk towards the teaching hospital, turn right past McDonalds, Starbucks, the Tanning Centre, and past the Operating Theatre Museum (avert gaze). We're both in really good spirits.

'That seems a bit cruel,' says Bruce, smiling and pointing at the pub sign over the road, swinging in the breeze.

'What do you mean?' I look up to see what has attracted his comment. 'Oh no, that *is* unfortunate.' The pub is called *The Bunch of Grapes.* I nudge Bruce playfully towards the doorway of the clinic. 'Try not to think about it honey, I'm sure he'll be gentle with you.'

'If only sperm were made in your elbow, or somewhere less embarrassing…'

'Come on. Let's get it over with.'

We climb the three brown-tiled steps up to the glass-panelled doorway, past the ambiguous signage, allowing a degree of anonymity to visitors. Immediately facing us through the external door is a notice welcoming us to the clinic, and directing us to the reception area through a second door to our right. Behind a counter sit two receptionists, a woman and a man, who greet us and ask for our names.

'Mr Lambert will be with you shortly,' says the woman. 'Please take a seat over there.' She's indicating the blue squishy chairs behind us. 'Water, tea or coffee is available from the machines; it's free of charge. Please help yourself. Were you able to bring your registration form for me?'

We had received the form and price lists the day after I'd made the appointments. It requested the usual: names, dates of birth, plus some quite detailed medical information, and what they termed in their literature as 'personal administrative information', apparently so that they can 'focus specifically on assessment and/or treatment issues during your first consultation'. Receiving it so quickly had been very reassuring.

We dutifully hand over the form. She checks that it has been completed properly. That's lovely, thank you.' We feel ridiculously pleased to have passed our 'entrance' exam.

The consultation

We are greeted in the waiting room by a tall, distinguished looking gentleman. We follow him just a few paces down the corridor into a consulting room. The walls display three framed collections of baby photographs. Some are smiling, some look bemused, one or two snapshots are of twins, but no doubt all are little blessings whose arrival has been welcomed and cherished by parents who have at last fulfilled a long-held dream. We get down to business.

'So, Mr Gallup,' says Mr Lambert. 'I have your results from Harley Street: you have high FSH levels. I believe that you have also had several negative sperm test results.'

'Yes, that's right,' Bruce replies. 'We were advised to come to a fertility centre; we understand that we may still have options.'

The consultant explains the reasons for a number of male factor problems, including a blockage in the outflow of sperm from the testes into the seminal fluid. There are a few reasons for this: some men are born without the main sperm-collecting ducts – the vas deferens or the epididymis; some may have sustained damage to the tubes at some point; others have undergone vasectomy, which has the same effect.

Mr Lambert continues: 'We can now look for sperm inside the scrotum and the testicular tissue. In some cases, if even a single sperm is found, it can be used to fertilize the female partner's egg. This is the process of ICSI – you may have heard about it. For men like yourself, this can be an option.'

'Okay. So what is the likelihood in my case of finding a small number of sperm?'

'Well, with your levels of FSH, I have to say that it is a little unlikely that we will be fortunate, but we shouldn't completely rule out the possibility of success.'

I want to know about the worse-case scenario: 'If there aren't any, what then?'

'Then I'm afraid that nothing more can be done.'

Bruce's thoughts turn to practical matters. 'How long will I have to take off work? I'm self-employed...'

'You may feel a little uncomfortable for a couple of days, but you should be back at work by next Wednesday.'

'What do you want to do?' I ask Bruce, afraid to push him to go through this undoubtedly painful, and potentially futile, procedure.

'Well, I need to find out, one way or the other, for my own peace of mind. I need to know what I'm dealing with here.' He seems determined to press ahead. Another question occurs to him: 'Our previous consultant told me that I had probably never produced sperm. Is there a way of knowing that for sure?'

'You can certainly discover, by means of a blood test, whether you have a part of your Y chromosome missing. That would be conclusive proof that you were born with this condition. If we do find any viable immature sperm, we would advise you to have the test.'

'Is that to do with the genes that Bruce would pass on to our child?'

'Yes, that's right. If you were to produce a male baby, then he would be in the same situation, regarding difficulties with sperm production, as his father.'

'And if there are none?' Bruce asks.

'Then whether you have the test or not is entirely up to you. Under those circumstances, the only way for you to have a child with genetic connections to one of you would be to use sperm from a donor. The sperm we use are very healthy, motile and numerous, so the problem does not arise.'

'Okay, thank you.'

'So,' says the consultant brightly, 'would you like to go ahead with the investigation tomorrow?'

'Yes I think so,' replies Bruce.

I'm so full of admiration for him; he's more confident than I would be, faced with all of this.

'If you would both like to go down to the day surgery unit on the lower ground floor when we finish, a nurse will be waiting there for you. She'll be able to give you a little more detail about the procedures and book you in for tomorrow.' Mr Lambert smiles, and shakes our hands.

As we leave the office, we're given a sheet of paper to take to Accounts. A quick glance tells us that the whole 'package' comes to just over £1000 – including an amount to cover freezing any sperm they find.

We pay our dues, then make our way out of the main reception and down the stairs. Here, we find ourselves entering a long rectangular room, which is rather dark. It contains six bed bays running the length of the room on the left; each of these has a green pull-across curtain for privacy. On the right-hand side are a couple of low circular coffee tables, each surrounded by four comfy chairs. Standing in welcoming anticipation next to a set of weighing scales is a nurse.

'Hello,' she chirps in a soft Irish accent. 'How are you doing? I'm Clodagh. You've seen Mr Lambert I take it?'

'Yes. He's lovely,' I reply.

'I'm Bruce. Hello. We've been told to come and see you.'

Well this is all very jolly. Perhaps this procedure isn't as bad as it sounds.

Clodagh weighs Bruce, asks him questions about smoking, for the benefit of the anaesthetist, and then explains the schedule for the following day.

'If you could stop eating and drinking from midnight please and be here to register at 11 tomorrow morning, Mr Lambert will carry out the PESA or TESE. Do you know what you're having done?'

'No, not really,' says Bruce. 'What's the difference?'

'Well, the PESA – percutaneous epididymal sperm aspiration – removes sperm from the storage duct with a very fine needle. TESE stands for testicular sperm extraction. It's not a savings plan!' We both giggle, as she's obviously heard that joke so many times before.

Clodagh explains that the specialist will remove any sperm he finds directly from the testes by taking several small tissue samples with medical clippers. She notices us wince at each other and quickly reassures us: 'Don't worry. You'll be given a local anaesthetic into the groin area so you won't feel a thing. An embryologist will be present, along with the anaesthetist, a nurse and the consultant. We analyse the samples straightaway under the microscope, so that if Mr Lambert finds any sperm, they can be frozen for use later on.'

'So do they keep them frozen while they start treatment with me?' I ask.

'Yes. You would have to be monitored through a monthly cycle, in a similar way to IVF, except that we have to use ICSI because the sperm aren't usually very motile...'

We are looking puzzled: 'Motile?'

'That means they are not very good swimmers.' She pauses to check that we've understood before outlining the process of prescribing drugs to make my ovaries produce more follicles than usual, which will, it is hoped, be fertilized by the sperm. Once the embryos reach six cells, they are placed back inside my womb. The good news is that if sufficient numbers of sperm are found and frozen, Bruce shouldn't have to go through the process for each of my cycles. They can be stored frozen for future use – not indefinitely, but long enough for our purposes. This sounds really hopeful. Clodagh has more information for us.

'The procedure will be over quite quickly, but we'll keep an eye on you for a couple of hours afterwards. If you could arrange a taxi Caroline, or bring a car, Bruce will need to be driven home – he won't feel comfortable enough to travel on public transport. Oh, and wear loose track-suit bottoms or something similar please.'

I see Bruce absorbing all the information about tomorrow, but my thoughts have leapt forward again to my part in all of this.

'Clodagh, I'm a bit overweight. Will this make any difference to my chance of conceiving?'

'It might lower your chances of success, and in terms of anaesthetics it is a little more expensive. Hop on the scales for me would you?'

I close my eyes and step up to be weighed, peeking at the dial as Clodagh says: 'Oh, that's not too bad. Just see if you can lose ten pounds or so.' *Ten pounds? That's a lot!*

The nurse must have seen my smile fading because she nudges me affectionately on the arm and makes a suggestion: 'Why not swap from red wine to white, or you'll just feel deprived. This is all stressful enough without having to go on a diet as well.'

I'm smiling again. What a nice woman. That's what I call a diet! With that, we say our 'au revoirs' and make our way out of the clinic, trying not to look at the pub sign on the way back to the underground.

★ ★ ★

Back at home, we realize that our next challenge is already on top of us: Bruce's mum, Alyson, is due to stay for the weekend, arriving tomorrow night. The visit has been arranged for a while, so we're going to have to tell her what has been going on. Nursing bruised anatomy, I'm sure Bruce won't feel much like acting the enthusiastic host.

Bruce picks up the phone and calls her.

There is no way of breaking the news gently or sliding seamlessly into the subject from talk of new colour schemes and whether we would like her to make any co-ordinating curtains. Bruce has to launch in, at an appropriate break in the conversation, and hope for the best.

'Mum, we'll come back to curtains in a moment, but the thing is that our situation tomorrow night has changed a little.' Pause. 'You see, Caro and I have been trying to start a family but nothing has happened. We've been having tests, and it appears that the problem lies with me. Um... I may be infertile.'

There seems to be no response for the moment. Bruce carries on.

'Tomorrow morning I'm having a surgical investigation to see if they can find any sperm; I'll probably be in bed recovering when you get here. We thought it best to let you know now, rather than give you a shock when you arrive.'

Bruce starts to pace the room whilst listening to her reply. He looks crestfallen. Eventually he speaks again.

'I see. Well, whatever you think is best. Bye now. See you soon.' He hangs up and turns to me: 'She's not coming.'

'Why not?'

'She thinks it would be better if she doesn't come. She doesn't want to intrude.'

'She's probably embarrassed. I'll call her back and talk to her if you like.'

'If you want to,' he says as he walks over to the TV remote control lying on the arm of our old sofa. He sits down and turns on the telly.

Over the 'phone to Alyson, I say that we would like to see her and that she won't be in the way. On the contrary, I could do with some family company, grateful for help with looking after Bruce. Her diffidence turns to warmth, and we agree that she'll arrive as planned the following evening.

The search for sperm

Each bay in the day surgery unit contains a trolley-bed and a chair. We were whisked downstairs as soon as we arrived and Bruce is now sporting one of those attractive backless cotton robes in this season's whites, blues and yellows. He is gasping for a cigarette and a coffee, but is remarkably good humoured considering he's done without since late last night. We've talked about him giving up – my pregnancy was going to be his target date – but he's under enough pressure at the moment, and if he has no sperm, it won't change anything anyway. We are last in line; there are five men ahead of him, presumably all having the same investigation. I'm surprised at the number and diversity of the couples here with us this morning, especially as this is a monthly clinic. A couple I estimate to be roughly in our age group are just disappearing through double doors at the end of the room, accompanied by two women and a man wearing operating theatre 'greens'. An older couple of middle-eastern appearance has just walked behind a cubicle curtain and an Asian couple is sitting in chairs at the other end of the room. I venture away from Bruce towards the coffee machine. A very young white girl, who looks to be barely out of her teens, is sitting by the machine, so close to it that it seems rude of me not to acknowledge her.

'There are a lot of us here aren't there,' I say. 'More than I expected.'

'Yes.' She smiles, but looks uncomfortable about entering into conversation, so I start to move away, back towards our cubicle.

'I hope it goes well for you,' I say, offering my support.

'Thank you. You too.'

I've changed my mind about the coffee, as it wouldn't be fair to Bruce. I sit down next to him. He's still quite cheery and seems really calm: 'Clodagh says that Mr Lambert will be in to see us in a minute.'

'This will all be worth it if they find sperm,' I say.

After about five more minutes, our consultant walks into the cubicle and smiles: 'Good morning. How are we today?'

'Well *I'm* fine,' I reply, instantly realizing how stupid and falsely 'breezy' I sound. I wince and feel guilty as my mind involuntarily makes a comparison with my trip to the vet last year taking our dog Barney to be neutered.

Mr Lambert turns to Bruce and begins talking to him softly. 'So, we'll soon take you down into the theatre at the end of this room. Clodagh and another nurse will bring you in to join the anaesthetist, our embryologist and me. Then, I'll give you a small injection of local anaesthetic in your groin and take biopsies of tissue from the testis.'

I love the way that doctors refer to 'the' part of the anatomy, as if separating from it being 'yours' will somehow make it hurt less.

'These samples will be analysed immediately to detect any sperm present. If we find any, we can freeze them for you. We'll have good news for you I hope.'

We concur and he leaves.

The surgeon must have done a couple of investigations before we arrived, because two bed bays at the far end of the room have their curtains part-closed.

'It's a bit disconcerting – being the last in line,' says Bruce. 'You'd better not tell me if anyone looks as if they are in pain.'

'I can't imagine women putting up with this "open queuing procedure" arrangement. It builds your anxiety a bit doesn't it?'

'Do you *mind*? I'm trying not to think about it.'

'Sorry.'

I poke my head out around the curtain, but see a pallid-faced man being pushed back into his bay from the theatre – and decide to retreat. His wife is shooting me a sympathetic half-smile.

Clodagh arrives to see us. 'Okay then?' *I wonder what they'd do if he said no?*

Off he goes. I'm not going in with him, although I was asked if I would like to – a bit too much for both of us, we decided. I wave him off, then grab a magazine from one of the tables and get myself that cup of coffee.

I've spent very little time in a medical environment. Except for my weekly visits to casualty with concussion after rugby as a teenager, I've never been in hospital – and rarely even go to the doctor. As I'm wheeled past the other 'victims' and their partners they look at me with slightly tense and sympathetic half-smiles. This strikes me as odd, as I feel okay! But they know what's to come, and I don't. I'm trying to cope by displaying an overemphasized sense of enthusiasm and cheeriness, but they are looking back at me, the look on their faces saying 'There there now (poor sod).'

Forty-five minutes later

'Hi. Welcome back. How was it?'

'Okay. A bit weird. The anaesthetist was very good. She obviously knew which bits of the procedure were the most painful. Just before one of those, she'd ask me a question about my life that required more than a one-word answer. She did her best to distract me, but that "clipping" noise as Mr Lambert took samples…that'll stay with me for quite some time. Actually, the worse part was the local anaesthetic injection, but at least it worked!' He smiles a slightly wicked smile, lifting the sheet covering his legs and lower body to reveal an article not dissimilar to a white cotton Satsuma bag, held in place by a tie around his waist. 'Oh, and sweetheart, I'm now the proud owner of a new item of rather sexy underwear.' He informs me that it is called a *scrotal support.* 'It's all the rage, so they tell me.'

I laugh, relieved at the fact that he still feels sufficiently okay to crack a joke. 'I'll ask Clodagh if you can have a hot drink, and then why don't you have a little doze, Casanova.' I lean across to kiss Bruce gently on the forehead and then go in search of our nurse.

Clodagh gives the go-ahead for a coffee, which I take in to Bruce. Just as I pull back the privacy curtain I overhear Mr Lambert talking to the couple in the next bay. It's the young girl I spoke to earlier and her partner: 'So it's good news for you. We found a few…enough, I think, to try to fertilize an egg. I am pleased for you.' I can hear 'smiling' agreement and 'happy' murmurs from the couple. 'You can leave in a little while. Let the nurses monitor your recovery. I will see you next month for a follow-up, so that we can plan a course of treatment for you both. All right then?' *Pause.* 'See you next month.' *Brilliant news. I'm sure we'll hear the same news very soon.*

I turn to Bruce. 'They found some sperm – for the couple next door…'

He replies gently, 'Yes, but during my procedure the doctor was passing tissue samples to the person at the microscope, who was checking them and then saying "No" each time. After each "no", Mr Lambert took another one.'

Mr Lambert walks in and pulls the curtain closed behind him. He puts his right hand gently on Bruce's leg, holding a document folder in the crook of his other elbow.

'I'm sorry, there were no sperm visible.'

My heart sinks. I can't smile any more.

He continues, 'But we will re-analyse the tissue in the laboratory. We may have missed one or two, let's hope we'll be lucky.'

He pats Bruce on the foot, wishes us a safe journey home and asks to see us next month for a follow-up appointment.

Clodagh comes in next to see how Bruce is feeling. She tells us that the lab will call us on Monday afternoon to give us the results of the second analysis.

In recovery, two hours after the procedure

Bruce is standing up gingerly and getting dressed. I'm passing his clothes to him from inside the temporary locker, so that he doesn't have to bend, but he seems fine.

'They're quite clever you know, Caro. I'm still numb from my groin down to my knees and I have painkillers for when the anaesthetic wears off,' he reassures me.

Clodagh brings in more advice sheets advising us on post-operative care: 'Watch out for any oozing, bleeding or swelling. If that happens, you must to go to your doctor immediately. Here's a list of the drugs you've had and the medical details of the procedure. If you have any problems, show this to your GP. Call us if you have any worries over the weekend; we're open on Sunday morning until one o'clock.'

We thank her and I go to bring the car round from the car park.

★ ★ ★

Bruce didn't feel the after-effects of the procedure during the journey home, but now he's in bed, in pain, and looking pallid. I'm sitting on the edge of the bed, trying not to put too much pressure on the bedclothes or to touch any tender parts accidentally. I'm helping him with painkillers. He hates taking them. Normally, he doesn't succumb unless he's in absolute agony.

The doorbell rings, Barney barks and I go downstairs to greet Bruce's mum. She's standing in the doorway, looking elegant and feminine in her trademark floral print skirt and simple, smart, pastel blouse. She has straight, shoulder-length hair, predominantly strawberry blonde, but now streaked with grey. She is ten years younger than my mother and, as a general rule, not as gregarious. She extends her arms towards me, drawing me into a welcome embrace as soon as my hand touches hers.

'How are you, my love? I'm sorry to hear your news. I know how much you wanted a family of your own.'

'Thanks for making the trip. Come on in.'

We go inside and she puts down her overnight bag in the hallway.

'Where's the wounded soldier then?'

'Upstairs in bed. Do you want to go up and see him?'

She follows me upstairs and into our bedroom.

'Hello there, Mum. Thanks for coming.' Bruce is sounding groggy, still looking as if a bus has hit him.

'Not feeling so good then?' she says.

'No, not really. Every time I try to stand up, I feel sick.'

I ask if he would like to eat something, not really expecting an answer in the positive. He declines, saying that he's going to go back to sleep. I take Alyson back downstairs so that we can begin getting supper ready. As we prepare the food together, we talk about her family.

She is one of four children, two girls and two boys, brought up on an award-winning dairy farm in the West Country. Whilst her brothers and sister all went into farming, Alyson had different ambitions. She excelled at science and passed maths, further maths and physics exams before leaving school. Eventually she became the only woman to be running an all-male department at the Ministry of Defence in the 1960s.

She excelled at motherhood too, leaving work to have three children, five years apart. So that she could make the most of family life, she set up her own nursery, a playgroup that became one of the most popular in the town.

'Did you always want a family?' I ask her.

'Yes, very much so. Having been brought up in the countryside, I always wanted my children to have the same idyllic childhood as I had: old fashioned… You know, lots of activities, games, nature walks and trips to the seaside.'

'From what Bruce tells me, you succeeded. He remembers the fun they had in the playgroup: making pictures with pasta, your cupboard at home full of craft materials and toys. I heard that you even made a rocket ship for Bruce in the back garden when Armstrong landed on the Moon.'

We laugh, but then Alyson says, 'You know it wasn't all plain sailing for me, don't you? I experienced the heartbreak of miscarriage, not once, but twice. I would have preferred my children to be closer in age than they were. Losing those two babies was unbearably painful. But in those days you weren't supposed to talk about it – just pull yourself together and get on with it…' She pauses briefly as we both stop what we're doing and then continues, 'Even though I do have children, I think I can understand how it must feel not to be able to have the child that you so desperately want.' She puts her hand on the back of mine, 'That's why I always encouraged you not to wait too long.'

I can feel a lump in my throat yet again. Alyson has told me about these painful experiences before, I know that she still feels the loss of those babies, even after all this time.

'I know, Alyson. I know you understand. I also really appreciate why you always wanted me to know what you'd been through so that I might not have to go through the agony myself.' Tears begin to fall down my face. 'The trouble is that I want *Bruce's* baby. I don't want anyone else's. Now I don't know what to do. The clinic are calling tomorrow afternoon, but it doesn't look like there's any hope.'

Alyson puts down the knife that she is using to chop vegetables. I grip mine even tighter. 'I can't bear this pain; my heart hurts. I feel lost, confused, and I don't know what to do to make it all right.'

Bruce appears in the kitchen doorway. 'Just thought I'd try to eat something, but I think I need to sit down.' He shuffles into the sitting room and moves towards the sofa.

My poor Bruce. There's no way he'll be back at work by Wednesday. It's going to be at least the weekend before he feels up to physical work again. I don't want to leave him to manage on his own; anyway, I'm sure that he can't. I need to think fast; contact my clients to re-arrange my week as well. We'll lose money if neither of us is working, but we've no choice right now. He needs time to recover.

Bruce eventually quells his queasiness and makes his way slowly back upstairs. Bruce and I have renamed the TESE a 'John Wayne-ectomy', in homage to Wayne's bandy gait. The evening passes quietly. Alyson washes up and I make a few calls re-scheduling meetings, citing Bruce's 'minor surgery'. I offer them assurances that it's nothing serious and that I will be able to keep on top of the workload from home. I feel slightly better once the pressure of maintaining appearances is lifted, at least for a while.

★ ★ ★

It's Monday afternoon, and we are alone in the house once more. The call comes from the laboratory confirming our worst fears – no sperm were found when the tissue samples were examined for the second time.

Bruce explains the starkness of the situation to me. 'Mr Lambert took 15 samples, more than usual, to be as thorough as possible. The fact that none was found in this amount of tissue means that I have probably never produced sperm.' He pauses, then looks at me, smiling: 'But guess what? There were no sperm to freeze, so we're getting a refund – about 250 quid. Not bad, eh?'

4

Chauffeur driven to Fertility Central

TESE follow-up appointment

The last four weeks have passed slowly; Bruce was in bed for most of the week following the operation. He returned to work because he had no choice, but had difficulty climbing ladders and had to employ an assistant, at his own cost, to do any lifting of paint tubs and spraying equipment for him.

This appointment is a formality really, as we already know what Mr Lambert is going to say: nothing else can be done. The only way for me to experience being pregnant and giving birth – for us to experience that together – is to use donor sperm. I'm contemplating the multi-coloured flecks in the blue waiting-room carpet when I hear a voice above my head: 'Mr Gallup please, and…'

A pair of highly polished brown leather shoes has appeared in my field of vision. I snap my gaze up away from the floor and meet Mr Lambert's smile with my own.

'Caroline,' I remind him, as I point at myself. We follow him through to the baby-pictures room. For us, the consultation is about one basic question: where do we go from here?

Mr Lambert gives us our options: 'If you wish, you could have a blood test to determine whether Bruce's condition is due to a chromosomal abnormality.'

Bruce looks at me. 'I don't see much point, do you? As I can't father children, nothing's going to be inherited, is it?'

'No, that's right,' confirms Mr Lambert.

I look away from Bruce now, then back at the consultant. *This can't be the end; I have to do something.* 'What could happen now – if we decide to go ahead with donor sperm?'

'You can make an appointment to see one of the other female fertility specialists straightaway to be assessed for donor insemination.'

Concluding the consultation, we both shake Mr Lambert's hand and walk out to reception, pausing at the accounts desk on our way through. Making an appointment for me to see someone seems simply the next tick on the 'To do' list. After all my original misgivings, I just want to get on with it; do the right thing for us. I want to get through whatever I need to do as quickly as possible so that we can get on with being parents.

We leave the building and descend into the underground, heading for home. Bruce seems remarkably upbeat and takes me by surprise – he appears to be more concerned about how I'm feeling than about his own disappointments, which must be enormous.

'Are you okay?' Bruce links arms with me, smiling.

'Yes. I mean I'm as disappointed as you must be, but at least this is all moving quite quickly.' *If I just keep pushing ahead, I'll soon be pregnant and this part will be over – this pain will be a memory.*

My first consultation

These chairs are becoming familiar. We already have a favourite place to sit in the waiting room, and Bruce has made it a point of principle each visit to take a boiled sweet from the selection at reception. We're back today for a series of appointments, beginning with an introduction to my new consultant. We've just seen the prices for various treatments, but they mean very little at the moment: IVF, ICSI, intra-uterine insemination (IUI), all with their associated costs of lab. work and drugs. If we have to have IVF, it will cost over £3000 for just one treatment. The same again each time if it doesn't work. I don't suppose it would have made any difference to the timing of our desire to have a family, but my being too old, at 38, to join the NHS waiting list is going to have a massive impact on our finances. Where are we going to find this sort of money?

Whatever we do, none of this will mean that I'm carrying Bruce's baby. So is it worth it?

'Miss Caroline Nicholson?'

I confirm my identity to the young woman standing in front of me. 'Please follow me,' she says.

This consultant, who has now introduced herself as Lisa di Martino, is a young Italian woman, wearing trendy spectacles, sporting cropped blond hair. She gestures us into a different room, a few steps further down the corridor. 'Please, call me Lisa.' *I like her; she's very positive.*

We all sit down around a desk and she opens our file, familiarizing herself with Bruce's results.

'You have to use donor sperm I think?' she commiserates, as she looks up at us over the top of her spectacles. 'Yes, I'm afraid so,' Bruce replies. The doctor looks back at me.

'What will happen now is that we'll give you a baseline scan to find out how your ovaries look – whether you have any problems – and then make an appointment for you to talk with the nurse and to choose donor characteristics. Afterwards you will return for blood tests and mandatory implications counselling before the start of your next cycle.'

'How long will it be before we actually get a go?' *That was rather clumsy – I made it sound like a fairground ride.*

'Depending on what we find today, plus the natural rhythm of your cycle, I should think about three to four weeks.'

'Okay.' I don't really know what to say now, I feel a bit numb. It seems a long time to wait. Dr Lisa stands up behind the desk. 'Shall we do the scan now?' She is indicating that we should leave the office. *Now? Now?*

I'm surprised at the speed and efficiency, but at least I don't have much time to be nervous.

'If you have no objection.' She smiles, still holding out her hand, gesturing towards the corridor. 'Don't worry, it's painless.'

'No, it's not that. I just wasn't expecting this to move so fast, but that's good. Thank you,' I reply.

Bruce and I follow her out of the room, turning left behind her, passing through a doorway marked 'Scanning Suite'. The room is gloomy and applying the term 'suite' is overstating it, given that there's only just enough space for the scanning machine, scanning operative and patient. Somewhat optimistically in my opinion, a chair has been squeezed next to the half-length medical couch. Bruce is following the doctor and me into the room, settling himself into the chair. It's a good job he's slim.

I spot a rather long, phallus-shaped instrument attached to the side of the monitor. Oh no, a vaginal scan. Now I feel even more embarrassed at the prospect of Bruce being present, but I don't want him to feel excluded, so I say nothing.

The doctor asks me to get undressed from below my waist. She turns away and begins discreetly shuffling paperwork on the other side of a scant privacy curtain. In position on the couch, knees bent up under a blanket, I mumble 'I'm ready' and she joins us from behind the curtain. She sits down by the machine and picks up the scanning probe.

'Now try to relax,' she says, as she skilfully and gently manoeuvres the probe into position inside my vagina. The movement is so deft, in fact, that I'm distracted from my embarrassment, becoming fascinated by the curved light-blue line to which Lisa now draws our attention: 'Here's the uterus you see,' pointing with the index finger of her free hand. Although I see the line, it bears no resemblance to any part of my anatomy that I might have imagined, but I'm in no position to argue. She measures the uterus lining to establish how far I have progressed through my monthly cycle, then moves the scanner into a new position. It doesn't hurt.

'Here is one ovary – the right one.'

'Wow,' Bruce pipes up. 'Now I *really* know you inside out.'

We all laugh and I feel less self-conscious.

'And here's the left ovary. You see these dark patches? These are the follicles beginning to grow. They are only a few millimetres at the moment. You're in the early part of your cycle. One of these follicles will grow faster than the others and become the dominant follicle. When you ovulate, it will be released into the fallopian tube.'

'I see,' I reply, still peering at the monitor. 'Fascinating.'

She removes the probe, apparently pleased with the state of my reproductive system.

'Well everything looks fine. If you'd like to get dressed now, I'll arrange for you to see the nurses. They will explain the procedures to you and answer any questions you have so far. Goodbye. Nice to meet you.'

I reach for my clothes and begin to get dressed. I'm so relieved that there are no problems. I had no idea that there were so many hurdles to leap.

Can I really accept a donor child into my life?

One aspect of the treatment is really bothering me: it's connected with the nature/nurture question. When our child is born, will I really feel that it is ours, or will I look into its eyes and only see a little stranger – the face of a donor I've never met? As our child grows, will I see characteristics and behaviour that I recognize from Bruce or me? Will I be able to share in the 'Boy, but he's stubborn; well he gets that from me' conversations? Will these anxieties be doubly strong for Bruce, who will have no genetic connection?

I often seek solace and relief from my mental torture by going for a walk in the park with Barney – he loves to chase a ball and retrieve it, never tiring of the game. Nowadays, however, even my breaks for fun and laughter have the capacity to turn into a trial of forbearance. A trip to the park almost always results in a friendly meeting with Fiona, one of our many dog-owning friends. It's a very open landscape, so even though I often feel less like talking these days, not to say 'Hello' and pass the time of day is completely out of character for me, and a signal to friends that something is wrong. Today is one of those days, as an acquaintance spots me walking down the avenue of cherry trees in blossom, next to the playground. Our respective dogs race away from us to sniff each other, tails wagging. As we come within earshot of each other, the dogs begin to play, circling around and around our legs.

'Hi Caroline! How are you and Bruce? Any news?' My heart sinks, not because I don't like Fiona, but because I don't know her very well, and now I regret mentioning on previous occasions that we are hoping to have a family, having moved into a larger house. This formerly innocent 'ice-breaker' has more wide-reaching implications now, and she has a look that tells me the sort of news she'd like to hear.

'Unfortunately, we're still having tests and nothing has happened on its own yet. The doctor thinks that there might be some problem.'

I'm getting accustomed to the fact that most people assume the problem lies with me, and don't think to enquire if this assumption is correct before offering advice.

'Don't worry,' says Fiona, waving her hand nonchalantly. 'A friend of mine had IVF and she had a lovely baby boy, first time – I'm sure you'll be *fine...*'

I don't want to embarrass her, or dismiss the well-meaning enquiry, because she obviously cares. Neither do I want to be disloyal to Bruce, who has asked me to keep his diagnosis a secret at the moment. So I just nod and smile. Inside I'm shouting, *It's not me, it's Bruce, and nothing I do will make any difference*, but how can I do anything but thank her for her support, agree that everything, 'I'm sure', will be 'fine'? We part and she walks on with her dog, happy to have helped, but I head for home more depressed than ever.

On the path near the exit from the park, I meet Barbara, who lightens my despondency with a little simple, compassionate listening. She lives just two roads away from me and I'm meeting her, running slightly late today, at the beginning of her walk with her mongrel, Harvey.

'Hi there! How are you today?' she asks.

Hesitantly, I decide to tell her the truth, because I know that she's also having fertility treatment. She's always been really open about her experiences: she has to use donor eggs. I've always felt sorry for her, but I never imagined I'd ever be in virtually the same boat.

'Well, I'm not pregnant yet Barbara and...we've just discovered there's a problem.'

'I see,' she replies gravely. 'Are you okay? Do you want to talk about it?'

I'm sure Bruce won't mind...she won't tell anyone. 'It seems Bruce has never produced sperm,' the words tumble out of my mouth, relieved to be liberated, 'so in order to have a child genetically connected to one of us, we have to use donor sperm. I'm frightened and I don't know whether I can do it or not.'

'Oh Caroline, I'm so sorry,' she empathizes. 'And what about you? Are you going to be all right?'

'I don't know yet. We haven't gone that far. I hope so, but to be honest, I can't get past having to use donor sperm.'

'Well, you know why I have to use donor eggs don't you?'

'Yes, you told me, endometriosis. But I don't really understand what that means.'

Barbara describes how tissue, similar to the lining of her uterus, grows 'ectopically', on the outside of her womb. This really messes with fertility. Basically, the tissue 'bleeds' like the lining of the uterus, but it can't escape from the body in the same way. So it becomes inflamed and engorged, causing cysts, internal scarring and terrible pain, which interfere with the function of the reproductive organs, bowel and bladder.

'Not all women have pain, and some are not infertile, but I certainly have a rotten time every month and spend a lot of time in bed,' she says.

'How awful! I had no idea it was so bad. Is there nothing that can be done to relieve it?'

'Well, some of the symptoms can be relieved with drugs, surgery, complementary therapies and nutrition, but there's no cure. Even with donor eggs, IVF hasn't worked so far. But we'll get there. I'm sure. We'll have a family somehow.'

I actually begin to feel fortunate it's donor sperm instead of eggs that we need, as Barbara has to wait anything up to two years for a suitable egg donor to be found, and then has to go through a cycle of IVF. She has to use a nasal spray to suppress her natural cycle, to bring her into line with the donor's ovulation and egg collection, and then do her own hormone injections, before the eggs are fertilized with her husband's sperm and the resulting embryos are implanted into her womb.

'Why do you persist if it's so awful?' I ask, trying not to seem judgemental about her choices.

'Well, it's more important than anything else to us, to be parents. If I can, I'd like to take every option available and try to conceive a baby genetically connected to one of us. That's why I put up with all the pain and inconvenience.' She looks up at the sky thoughtfully. 'I do freak out a little with the embryo transfer – I'm wiser now and ask for a sedative beforehand – it's the anticipation of pain rather than any terrible reality.'

I make a mental note to speak up if I'm uncomfortable with anything that's done to me in the forthcoming weeks.

Barbara continues, 'But, I don't remember if I told you, I'm adopted and so is my brother, so ultimately if this doesn't work out, Pete and I'll be happy to adopt – anything to have a family.'

'Goodness Barbara, I take my hat off to you; you're so resilient, so strong. I could never do what you've done – injections I mean.'

'Well, they can't be helped. My cycle has to match the donor's, and the lining of my uterus has to be "bumped up" in thickness to help the embryos implant. I try not to think about it if I can help it. I just block it out as best I can and get on with it. You develop a stoicism I suppose – you *have* to focus on a positive outcome.'

What if this doesn't work? Even if it does, am I kidding myself?

'If I can never have *Bruce's* baby – I love him so much. I'm not sure that this is what I want to do.'

The dogs are getting bored: Barney has smelt some mouldy bread just in reach at the end of his extendable lead and he's tucking into it with gusto.

Harvey has started to bark incessantly; Barbara scolds her pet: 'All right, all right, be quiet will you, we're going.'

She begins to walk away, barely keeping him to heel, but then stops, turns and offers me a lifeline: 'Well, if you need to talk, you know I'm available. I had a friend who was further through her own treatment when I started. It really helped. She found a support organization for me to contact. It won't be relevant for you, but there are loads of them out there. Have a look on the Internet. I can drop round with a few of our old magazines from donor support organizations if you like.'

'That'd be great. Thanks.' I turn my attention to my own greedy hound, persuading him to stop gobbling the mouldy bread by giving him a tastier treat from my pocket.

As I attach the lead to his collar, I wish Barbara well. 'Good luck with your next cycle.'

'And good luck with making the right decision for you and Bruce,' she replies. 'Don't be persuaded into doing something you really don't want to do. It's a tough old road ahead of you. Promise me you'll only do what you feel is right for you?'

'Yes. Absolutely,' I promise as I walk away.

I did manage to keep my promise to Barbara during the course of my treatment, but my increasing desperation meant that I came to consider – and agree to – options that I would have dismissed out of hand when we had our conversation.

The nurses talk

We're back at the clinic, back in the baby-pictures room where we first met Mr Lambert. Sitting in front of us are two smiling young women who introduce themselves as Brenda and Ruth.

'Hello. Come in. Take a seat.' Brenda is friendly, has a kind, slightly freckled face, brown shoulder-length hair and pale-blue eyes. She explains that Ruth would like to observe the session as part of her training, if we don't object. We agree, so Brenda opens the document folder lying on the desk in front of her. My name is written on the cover in large black letters.

'Now then, first things first,' she says. 'From now on, please give *your* name when you ring for anything Caroline, as we file everything under the female patient's name.'

'I'm surplus to requirements am I? I can take a hint,' jokes Bruce.

'Well we *do* hope not. You will be the father after all won't you? You can be involved with any part of Caroline's treatment. There's no restriction. You can be together as much or as little as you choose.'

'So he can be with me when I have the insemination?'

'Yes, and for all the examinations if you want – there's no need to be separated at all. It's up to you.' She looks down again at my notes. 'Now, you'll be having IUI to start with – intra-uterine insemination with donor sperm. This technique uses your natural cycle, placing the donor sperm directly into your uterus. Normally there are two potential barriers to achieving fertilization: one is the vagina, where sperm can't survive very long; and the second is the cervix. In IUI, by injecting the sperm directly into the uterus, we by-pass those two barriers.'

'You mean they're chauffeur driven to Fertility Central?' The image of a stretch limo flashes into my head – sperm in sunglasses, sipping Margaritas and giving each other 'high fives'.

'Yes,' Brenda laughs. 'Not quite in a Rolls Royce though. The sperm are inserted from a syringe, through a catheter. That way, we can be sure there's no problem between the seminal fluid and cervical mucus. For some couples the sperm can't survive because of incompatibility with vaginal fluids.'

'Goodness,' I say, 'it's a wonder anyone manages to get pregnant naturally. I had no idea it was fraught with such difficulties.' I'm more fascinated than nervous at the moment. This is beginning to feel like an acceptable option to me – not exactly natural, but the next best thing if we can't conceive a baby together.

Bruce takes my hand as Brenda continues to explain that they first have to test hormone levels to check my current fertility level, as well as screen my blood to measure the effectiveness of the rubella (German measles) jab I received many years ago at school.

'We also test for genetic problems such as cystic fibrosis, sexually transmitted infections like Chlamydia, and something called cytomegalovirus (CMV for short),' she explains. 'Most people have contracted CMV at some stage and, although for an adult it has no symptoms and no dangerous implications, it *can* cause problems for a foetus. In the case of a CMV-positive recipient, the donor can be either CMV positive or negative, but because of the current donor shortage, clinics usually match a

CMV-positive recipient with a CMV-positive donor. If the recipient is CMV negative, clinics have to find a CMV-negative match.'

'I'm glad that you're testing for Chlamydia,' I say. 'I've seen a number of news items on the television about the increase in infections. There are no symptoms, but it can seriously affect fertility – is that right?'

'Yes. If a woman has unprotected sex with a number of partners, the risk of being infected increases. Not all women have symptoms, but in up to 40 per cent of those that do become infected and don't get treated, the infection spreads into the uterus or fallopian tubes. It can damage the tubes or cause a potentially fatal ectopic pregnancy.' Brenda tells us that health awareness campaigns are encouraging all sexually active young women over the age of 25 to be screened, but the message is not catching on quickly enough.

'I was sexually active just before the AIDS scare,' I remember. 'I was on the contraceptive pill from the age of 19. I wasn't by any standards promiscuous, but do you think there's a real risk of me having it?'

'Let's hope not,' replies Brenda, not allaying my panic at all. Unlike Bruce, I may have done something stupid that prevents this working.

Brenda turns a page in my file, pen poised over an empty chart, and begins filling in my name at the top.

'The only other thing you'll need to do for us prior to your first treatment is establish at what point in your cycle you have your LH surge – that stands for luteinizing hormone. It tells us when, or *if*, you ovulate. If you don't, then IUI isn't an option. If you do, we need to know when so that we can introduce the sperm at the optimum time for fertilization. We'll be asking you to start testing as soon as possible. Do you know the date of your last period?'

'About a week ago.'

'So you're now at about day seven?'

'Seven, eight or nine – I'm not sure.'

Brenda asks me to start testing the following day. A surge happens mid-cycle – 24 to 36 hours before ovulation. The pituitary gland produces the surge of LH, triggering your ovaries to release an egg from the most developed follicle. The egg lives for 24 to 36 hours, and the sperm for two to five days. Insemination is done the day after the surge so that the sperm and egg have the greatest chance of finding each other.

'Do I have to come here to test?' I ask, although I'm nearly at information overload now.

I thought my biology classes at school were serving me well until I walked into this. How little knowledge I had. How lucky are parents who just conceive without knowing all of this.

'No. Well, you *can* if you don't feel confident about using a kit at home, but you seem a capable woman and it's very simple. It's very similar to a pregnancy testing kit – you pee on a stick in the same way and then wait to see blue lines in the little windows. Otherwise you'll spend a lot of time and money coming here every morning.'

I say that I'll buy a Clearplan ovulation testing kit from the chemist on the way home.

'Good. Now, if you're not too overwhelmed, I can tell you what happens after the tests are complete, or would you like to leave it there for today?'

'Let's have all the information please,' says Bruce. 'Bring it on,' he grins.

'Okay,' says Brenda. 'Once all these tests are complete, you'll come in to select characteristics. We'll explain more to you then, but let me tell you a little about how we select our donors. The men are volunteers...'

'Can you imagine the Press Gang technique if they weren't?' Bruce interrupts playfully.

I thump him gently on the arm, 'Bruce!'

'Oh my goodness,' laughs Brenda. 'Let's move swiftly on shall we?'

She goes on to explain the various sources of donor recruitment: medical schools, local colleges and businesses. In countries where donor anonymity has been removed, the profile has changed, moving from young, single students to older, family men in stable relationships.

'The most important criteria are that the donors are healthy men, below the age of 45, with a good motile sperm count. The sperm are washed as well, as a safety precaution, as most of the viral nasties, like HIV [human immunodeficiency virus] – the virus causing AIDS [acquired immunodeficiency syndrome] – and many sexually transmitted infections, are all held in the seminal fluid.'

'What motivates someone to donate?' I ask.

'Well, we don't really know, but there must be a certain amount of altruism in their motives, especially now that the anonymity of donors has been removed in a lot of countries.'

She outlines the tests the donors have to go through in order to be accepted. We're reassured, but surprised, that they're quite intrusive. 'Donors are tested more rigorously: we test for HIV/AIDS; sexually transmitted diseases and minor infections; hepatitis B and C as well as Chlamydia and CMV. We can also screen for any ethnically specific or hereditary conditions like sickle-cell anaemia, thalassaemia and Tay-Sachs disease. The sperm sample is quarantined for six months, to make sure that HIV is not present and to ensure that it survives the freeze/thawing procedure. The potential donors are asked about their sexual activity, and promiscuous men are not accepted. They have to refrain from intercourse prior to giving a donation to make sure that there are plenty of sperm.'

'It makes you grateful that they're prepared to donate at all to help couples like us,' I say.

Bruce asks, 'What do we do about the new anonymity laws – obviously it will affect me as the non-biological father?'

Poor Bruce, how will we cope if our child rejects him as 'Dad' at some stage, knowing that his biological father is another man? I don't want him to feel sidelined, but he must be seeing that as a very real possibility.

'The counselling session will cover all of that for you,' replies our nurse. 'Our counsellors are more informed about that side of things. Implications counselling is mandatory I'm afraid. Have you made your appointment yet?'

'We haven't, but we will – on our way out.'

Brenda places the pen on the desk, but seems in no hurry to close down our lines of communication: 'Now, do you have any other questions on the medical side?'

'Yes. What happens now? There's so much to take in, I've forgotten.'

'You've had your scan, so now you need to begin testing at home for your surge, and give us a call when you've had it. After your implications counselling, come back to us to choose characteristics, and then it's just a matter of waiting for your next menstrual cycle to start. Call us on the first day and we'll book you in.'

'So within a couple of months, I could be pregnant?'

'Yes, let's hope so.'

As we get up to leave, Brenda shakes our hands. 'Well good luck. We'll see you again very soon.'

We leave the room, still holding hands until we reach reception. We make the next two appointments and pay for this last batch – another £90 for the scan. Bruce grabs a sweet and we decide to go for a drink to celebrate. We veer away from the portals of the Bunch of Grapes in favour of finding a more sympathetically named hostelry around the corner.

5

'And how do you feel about that?'

Implications counselling

Although our experiences so far have been very positive, I find our circumstances very depressing. I wanted the 'make love, make a baby' experience. I wanted to miss a period, do a private pregnancy test, cook a special meal for Bruce and see his face light up as I reveal our exciting news: 'Darling, you're going to be a father.' But instead, as I understand it, this process of conceiving our child will be all about being in a room with bright lighting, sterile medical equipment, a test tube full of sperm and a nurse inseminating me with a catheter. Bruce can choose to be with me if that's what we want, but it won't make a difference to the procedure if he decides to wait outside. This is a long, *long* way from being an expression of love between two people. The disappointment is hard to deal with.

Our counsellor is called Steven. Initially I feel slightly awkward, but his kind smile and easy confidence ease my anxiety.

We're sitting in a primrose-painted room, square, with no windows. It has a relaxing atmosphere, helped by soft light emanating from conical wall lights fixed either side of an abstract painting. There is a large pot plant to the left of two blue, low-backed easy chairs. Steven sits opposite, in an identical chair, next to a low desk, where he has placed a document folder, writing pad and discreet clock.

'Now then,' says Steven, 'first things first. Although at this stage counselling is mandatory, this is an informal session. If you've read the Human Fertilisation and Embryology Authority's guide to infertility, you'll have seen that all clinics licensed by the HFEA offer implications counselling before you consent to treatment.'

Much to Bruce's irritation, we know that the HFEA consider this counselling to be essential, particularly for couples like us using donor gametes.

'I am legally bound to impart certain information to you,' says Steven. 'But otherwise this session gives us the opportunity to talk about anything at all. It's important that you understand exactly what's involved in conceiving a donor child, and how it might affect you. Our sessions are confidential, although I will take notes from time to time. I like to keep things as informal as possible, so please call me Steve. Can I call you Bruce and Caroline?'

'Yes, of course, that's fine. Where do we begin?' I ask.

'As I said, this is *your* session,' he emphasizes, making an open, inviting gesture, then resting his hands on his knees and inclining forward in his seat.

Bruce coughs uncomfortably into his loosely curled fist. This isn't something he would enter into, given the choice. If Bruce has a problem, he tends to keep it to himself, usually mulling it over whilst fixing something on the car or making something for our home. Conversely, I prefer to talk things through with him or my friends. I had bereavement counselling a couple of years ago, following the death of my father, which I found very helpful. I'm perfectly comfortable talking to a professional. To me, it's not daunting or intrusive. In fact, I've been looking forward to it.

I decide to remain quiet, giving Bruce a chance to speak, but he doesn't, so Steve breaks the ice.

'Obviously you've been through a great deal already, so can I ask how you are coming to terms with your diagnosis?'

Bruce looks at me, so I decide to step in with a question: 'How common is our problem?'

'You're referring to azoospermia?'

'That's the official name for it then?' asks Bruce.

'Yes,' Steve replies. 'Well let me see. I've spoken to six couples today and three of the male partners, including you, are azoospermic, so it's not that unusual I'm afraid. How do you feel about it?'

'Well, it is what it is I suppose,' Bruce replies pragmatically. 'It had never crossed my mind that I may not be able to have my own children, but at the same time it didn't really come as a surprise. I know that sounds strange.' Bruce smiles at Steve for the first time as he continues, 'I think we're okay about it now – now that the initial shock and the unhelpful way in which our GP dealt with it have faded a little.'

'Yes, I'm afraid I do hear some horror stories about general practitioners,' Steve interjects. 'You know that you're perfectly at liberty to change your GP if you're really unhappy. You could look for someone with a special interest in fertility.'

'We may well do that at some point,' continues Bruce, 'although a locum we saw said that she had some expert knowledge, but it didn't help us in the long run. I don't suppose she could have known that I'm...azoospermic did you say?'

'That's right,' replies Steve.

I feel a flush of rage as the two men calmly discuss our circumstances. How can Bruce be so calm? I can't hold back my anger any longer and burst out, 'Actually I'm *furious* with this situation. I wanted *Bruce's* baby. Is there absolutely *nothing* that can be done?'

'For azoospermia? No, not at the present time, I'm afraid.' Steve's hands move apart, palms turning up to the ceiling, and his eyes widen and calmly meet my angry stare. He offers more guidance: 'If you like, in addition to our sessions I can pass on details of support networks you can contact. There's a very good one called the Donor Conception Network. The founders are a couple who have three donor-conceived children. They are all now grown up.'

Steve pauses and checks that I have no need to say any more for the moment. I can't think of any more that I want to say. I just want to get out of here – to have a chance to talk to Bruce alone.

The counsellor changes tack to talk about my impending treatment. 'Now, Caroline, you haven't had any tests yet, but how do you feel about the whole issue of donor gametes?'

'Gametes?' I ask.

'It's the general term we use to refer to donor egg or sperm.'

'Eggs? But I'm fertile; my tests came back normal. I have my own eggs, so I'll be all right won't I?'

'Oh yes, I'm sure you will be. But some patients have to, or choose to, use both if there are both male and female factor issues.'

I still don't know what he means, but this potential scenario has tickled my sense of humour, and my imagination has involuntarily conjured up a surreal image, making me laugh aloud.

'Well, if that's the case for me, you might as well order a thermal box from Marks and Spencer and I'll watch the baby gestate in the corner of our living room. What's the point of using donors for both?'

'Well, some women are very clear that they want the birth experience...'

Only now, years later, do I understand that Steve probably wanted to assess my views on pregnancy and birth and to see whether or not this was something I desperately wanted, but at that stage it went completely over my head.

As I continue giggling, he begins to laugh *with* me, and obviously thinks better of pursuing this line of discussion. But it's served to break the ice, allowing us to relax. He continues.

'As I explained at the beginning of our session, as well as this being a chance to explore your feelings and concerns, I need to tell you about the legal implications of using donor sperm. Are you aware of the impending law change removing the right of donors to anonymity?'

'Only from the television and newspapers. How will it affect us?' asks Bruce.

Steve explains. 'At the moment, any child already living, who was conceived by donor gametes, does not have the right to know from whom those gametes came. However, children conceived after the first of April 2005 will have the right to request detailed, identifying information about their donor once they reach the age of 18. The law change benefits them by granting them the same rights to information about their origins as adopted children. In New Zealand, Australia, Denmark and the Netherlands the law changed some time ago. Here in the UK, this year and next year, you'll find yourselves in a transition period. When you choose donor characteristics you'll only have access to sufficient information with which to choose your donor. But I would suggest that, being so close to the law change, you need to give serious consideration to whether or not you are going to tell your children how they were conceived.'

'How do we even begin to make that decision?' I ask.

'Well, the Donor Conception Network have brought out quite a lot of information – advice sheets based on real experiences, and I believe they have a DVD called *Telling and Talking*.'

Steve also mentioned that in 1996 the Australian Donor Conception Support Group held a forum. As a result, quite a bit of research is available on the views of donor offspring in their teens and early adulthood. The general view appears to be that it is better to tell donor-conceived children of their origins as soon as possible. Children who had been told in later years testified at the forum that they grew up with a sense that something was being hidden, which made them feel uneasy and somehow different. Steve made the very practical point that it's very, very hard to destroy every piece of documentation relating to insemination treatment, or for it to remain entirely confidential. If our child were to stumble across any information unwittingly, we could see how this could cause a great deal of upset for our family.

This all seems to be a huge amount to think about. We've been catapulted into some sort of alien world, so far removed from our normal lives that I am finding it difficult to believe that all this applies to us and to something as simple as trying to have a baby.

I can't quite organize my thoughts to say very much to Steve, but using donor sperm and adoption seem to be two different things to me. This child will be the product of our relationship, not any other. I understand the right of children to know where they came from, but I'll be the only father our children will ever know, won't I?

'And if we decide not to tell?' asks Bruce.

'Well,' replies Steve, looking at him, 'of course there's no way of obtaining the views of children who have never been told.'

I imagine us sitting with our teenage children: 'Your father and I have something to tell you…'

Steve's voice interrupts my thoughts. 'If you decide that you won't want to tell your child, perhaps you should consider keeping this treatment secret from your friends and family.'

Steve makes the point that it's very awkward if Aunty Flora or Grandad has been told and then you find yourself torn because your relatives feel that the child should know as well. On a medical, rather than a social, level, if the child ever needs donor material for transplant, or requires medical attention for a hereditary condition, it's very valuable to be able to source genetically connected individuals, for everyone's benefit, including the donor.

'It's a little late for that I'm afraid. Our mothers already know there's a problem with us having our own children,' I say.

Steve clears his throat: 'Okay then. You can get back to me any time if you need more advice. Sorry to push on, but we're running out of time today I'm afraid. Don't worry, if we need another session, I'll arrange it. There'll be no extra charge. I need to cover consents and contracts with you. Is that okay?'

Steve hands us consent forms. We must sign one each before we can proceed with treatment.

'Before any assisted conception treatment can begin, both parties must give written consent. There are three types of consent involved in HFEA-licensed treatment: consent to your treatment – no different from the form you have to sign for other medical procedures; consent to disclosure of information...'

'What information is disclosed and to whom please?' I interrupt. 'I thought we had the choice not to tell anyone?'

'Yes you do, but it's a good idea to inform your GP of your treatment, and sometimes GPs can help you by ordering in drugs for your cycles. The clinics can decide whether or not to contact GPs, but they prefer to let them know that their patients are having treatment, just in case there are problems or anything in the health records that the clinics should be aware of. If you decide not to let us have the contact details, we would hold a case conference to decide if treatment should go ahead, although no-one would be able to withhold approval unreasonably.'

'You're joking!' I exclaim. 'Our doctor, who hardly knows us, has an input into our decision to be parents! Not only does she have very little knowledge of this treatment, but I've only seen her for an ear infection and a bad back; Bruce has seen her once to register and once to be told he's infertile.'

'It's more to prevent known paedophiles or people with children already on an "at risk" register slipping through the net.'

'I see,' I reply. 'Well good luck. She hasn't been that helpful so far – it's down to my gynaecologist that we found any information at all and ended up here.'

Treading gingerly, the counsellor begins to speak again.

'And...the third type of consent is for the use and storage of eggs – not applicable in your case – but also of any embryos produced if you have IVF.'

Bruce hands me his consent form, which I fold and push into my handbag, together with my own. Steve looks down at his notes, then up at us.

'Sorry, not much more to get through now,' he smiles. 'You're not married are you?'

We shake our heads and he continues.

'So you will also have to arrange a contract giving Bruce paternal rights over the baby. If you are unmarried, the father's name on the birth certificate will remain blank.'

'But that's *terrible*,' I blurt out. 'How insulting!'

'That's the law as I understand it,' replies Steve.

I turn to look at Bruce, who is frowning at Steve. I have an idea: 'Or we could just get married?'

Bruce is still looking at Steve, but Steve is looking from one to the other of us, as if watching a rapid-fire tennis rally, searching, I assume, for any conflict. After all, this is the first time he's met us.

'Is this a new idea, Bruce?' he asks.

Bruce looks surprised, then concerned, and then smiles. 'Oh no, we've talked about it for years. We've just never got round to doing it,' he replies, without looking in my direction.

How amazingly matter of fact of him. Any conversations we've had about marriage in the past have been at my instigation. I've always thought that he was against the idea. If he means it, it would be a dream come true.

The counselling session over, we make our way home. Although we are still holding hands and excitedly discussing the prospect of having a family, a fundamental difference in our responses is emerging. Bruce is very upbeat and encouraging. Whilst happily discussing the wonderful opportunities available to us and trying to probe a little deeper into Bruce's apparent amenability to a wedding, in reality I feel more like the girl from the 1970s horror movie *The Exorcist*: my head is spinning and a silent scream is convulsing from the depths of my gut. Whenever I think about donor sperm, I feel nauseous and as if something deep in my heart just died. My grieving process had begun, although I didn't realize it at the time.

What shall we tell our child?

Bruce switches on the television to catch the latest news. He settles down on the sofa with Barney, a beer and a cigarette.

'Hi honey. You all right?' I ask. He looks tired but I need to talk about my doubts with him. I begin the conversation as gently as I can. 'Are you okay with this my lovely – the donor sperm? It doesn't seem to be an issue with you. Somehow I would have expected you to have reservations.'

'Yes. I'm okay. Honestly,' he says. He drags on a roll-up and then exhales the smoke, rolling the head of the cigarette around the edge of the ashtray in front of him.

'I know that I said I couldn't do it,' I moot. 'But if you think it's the right thing to do, I'm beginning to I feel that I *can* go ahead with this treatment. I have to admit, when we first found out, I was strangely relieved that it was all so conclusive – no grey areas – and I suppose I didn't expect you to want to try anything else, but I can see that you're all for it now.'

'Well, obviously it's not *ideal*, but I don't see why being infertile should prevent me becoming a father. That seems a *ridiculous* reason to stop.' He looks at me questioningly. 'Does that sound stupid?'

'No, not at all. You'd make a brilliant father; I thought that when we first met.'

Bruce sits next to me on the sofa and Barney nestles in between us, sighing and resting his head on Bruce's lap.

'I was wondering what do you feel about the "To tell or not to tell" question that Steve mentioned. If we do this thing, what do you want to do about telling the child...about being conceived by donor sperm?'

'My instinct is to tell, to be honest, even though it will be tough. For one thing, it removes any ammunition in the troublesome teenage years – I can just hear that phrase "You can't tell *me* what to do, because you're not my real father." At least I'd have the retort "You've always known that. Just remember that I've been your *only* father. I've cuddled you, provided your food, changed your nappies, picked you up when you fell and helped you with your homework."' He finishes his fantasy scenario, looking down at the coffee table as he peels the next column of ash from the end of the cigarette into the ashtray. 'And I much prefer this option to adoption.'

I offer to look for information on the Donor Support Network recommended by Steve and go into the office to turn on the computer.

A fruitful search on the Web informs me that the support group was started in 1993 by a group of families who had all chosen to be open with their children about their origins. Clicking through to the *Planning a Family* section provides three documents written by two of the founding members – Olivia and Walter Merricks. I print off the papers and bring them into the living room. They're in the form of a letter about donor insemination from Walter to would-be DI dads, and a letter from Olivia to would-be DI mums, plus some information to DI parents about talking and telling. I scan the pages, summarizing the information for Bruce, reassuring myself at the same time.

'Olivia seems to have felt exactly as I do about not being able to have her husband's child. According to her all my crying can be attributed to grief and bereavement. It all makes sense to me. *And* they had an insensitive GP.'

I begin to read out sections of feelings experienced by patients.

'"Shock, despair, anger, disappointment, deep sadness (at not being able to have a loved partner's child), protectiveness (towards partner…) are all part of the see-sawing emotions women are likely to go through." She also points out that, because of my age, time may be running out for me in terms of fertility, so now there's the added pressure of not being able to take time to adjust to the news or the treatment.'

'What does the letter to DI dads say?' asks Bruce, leaning towards me to read over my shoulder. 'Anything useful?'

'Well, it mentions your fears about telling people, but says that they are generally unfounded. Apparently, if you have good friends and you pick the right time to tell them about your difficulties, most people feel privileged to be in on such a private piece of news. There's also some helpful stuff about how things worked out for them; they have a girl and a boy, both from different donors.'

'Did they suffer the "you're not my dad" taunts?'

'Apparently not. Look, it's here: it hasn't happened to them, or any other DI family they know. Walter thinks this is because his kids know that he's not ashamed of his infertility, and therefore that saying something like that won't press any of his buttons. Listen: "We all know I'm not genetically related to them, but I'm not ashamed of my infertility and they know it. They absolutely accept me as father, partly because they clearly haven't got another one, and partly because I have all the responsibilities and authority that go with the role of being their father – genes don't tell us how to love."'

'That's true,' Bruce nods. He seems reassured, and gets up and heads for the kitchen. 'What do you want for supper?'

I carry on reading. 'I don't mind, honey. Whatever you feel like cooking; you're the expert. Anything's fine.'

I'm not really concentrating on Bruce's enquiry, being somewhat distracted by a note of caution from Walter and Olivia; it's something that hasn't really occurred to me. I shout out to Bruce.

'They do warn that when the baby's born, you have to be ready, pretty much in the delivery room, for the "who does he or she look like?" question.'

'Well yes, I suppose you do,' Bruce replies, with his head still in the fridge. 'How do they suggest dealing with that?'

'Well it's one of the reasons that they recommend that people know what you're doing right from the outset. Otherwise the choice is to dismiss remarks, or just say that the baby looks like the mother and try to move on as fast as possible.'

Bruce has walked back into the room carrying a tray of our favourite snacks.

'So, we're going to tell?'

'Yes, I think so, don't you? I've never been any good at keeping secrets. The Donor Conception Network recommend telling the child as soon as possible – even before they can fully understand what you are saying – it helps to practise the words apparently.'

'They also advise involving teachers and close friends: if the children mention their origins when their parents aren't around, it can be explained with a minimum of fuss, without the children feeling different from their peers. I'm trying to absorb exactly what we are taking on. The implications are far reaching – I had no idea.'

I put down the sheets of paper, turning to face Bruce, who is dipping a sliver of pitta bread into a pot of houmous. He looks up, probably sensing that I'm going to make a proposal for action.

'So…?' he says, waving the pitta out to one side. 'You look as if you want something to happen, honey. Tell me your thoughts.'

'Sooo…how about making a start? How about telling your father and your sisters what's going on? Our mums already know. I'm sure they'll keep quiet if we ask them to, but it's not fair that they have all the pressure of being the only ones in the family who know.'

'Yes, okay. I'll sleep on it. I just need a little time to mull it over, to see if I'm ready to "take it by the balls" so to speak.' He smiles his cheeky smile before taking a quick swig of beer. 'No pun intended,' he says, putting the glass thoughtfully back down on the table. 'I mean that I want to have my answers ready.'

'Come here, my lovely man.' I put my arms around him, enveloping him in a big bear hug finishing with a kiss.

The decision to tell our child of its origins was right for us. We felt that it was our responsibility to give our baby the most straightforward start in life that we could. We are not much good at being secretive, and we suspect that we'll need the support of our friends more than ever when we face our difficult journey.

The increase in health tourism in the past few years has meant that parents can still opt to receive sperm from an anonymous donor despite the law change in the UK, but whether anonymity for donors stays in place, or is removed, the question to tell or not to tell never actually changes.

An exciting proposal

Sunlight is streaming into the extension at the back of the house, where Bruce and I sit at weekends, talking out problems or making plans. Despite the reassurances found in the Donor Conception Network literature and from the counsellor, I had another sleepless night. I didn't want to disturb Bruce by tossing and turning, so I spent most of the night downstairs watching trashy television, trying to make sense of my feelings. Grief overtakes anger and back again, but both make me cry. This morning, I feel like a wrung-out dishcloth. Bruce, on the other hand, seems buoyant. He isn't working today, and I have no client meetings until this afternoon, giving us the chance to talk, to check through the decisions made yesterday. I need reassurance that he's happy for me to go ahead with treatment.

'Are you sure?' *Part of me wants him to say he'll love me either way, but he seems totally focused on this option.*

'Yes. I'm surprised, but I'm fine,' he replies. 'As I said last night, I feel that my being infertile is not a good enough reason not to be a father'

I think he's being very brave and tell him so. It's me who needs to summon up courage it seems. I change the subject.

'I was shocked by your reaction to my suggestion of marriage. I never expected you to say that we should. I didn't know that we had always intended to…'

'Well I thought we had, but maybe I didn't get around to telling you. Sorry, lady,' he grins. Barney is sitting at his feet; tail wagging, waiting for the go-ahead to jump up on his lap for a cuddle. 'Up you come then, Puppy.'

It feels right to create some good omens, make good causes – to get the universal forces working in our favour. I believe in cause and effect, so by making the right causes to welcome our child into the world we will encourage the effect that we want – successful insemination. As long as we do everything we possibly can by working hard, staying healthy, filling our hearts with love for each other and our child, surely our prayers will be answered. I assumed that the child I visualized whilst chanting was a child conceived naturally by Bruce and me, but who knows, I could have been wrong. He was our child and he still can be, even if I do have to use a donor.

'So did you mean it?' I ask Bruce. 'Do you really want to get married?'

If he does, not only will our wedding be an oasis amidst all this difficulty, but it will also give me the perfect way to prove to Bruce that I love him, no matter what, and that his diagnosis has made no difference at all to my feelings for him.

'Yes, why not?' he says, grinning at me. 'I feel really close to you after all this. It really feels right to do this now.'

'We could get married at the Buddhist centre, if that's okay with you?'

'Yes, why not – as long as it's legal,' he jokes. Prior to a UK law change allowing the legal contracting words to be included within a Buddhist ceremony, couples had to marry in a registry office, then hold a separate religious occasion.

I get up out of my chair, straightening my dressing gown, and walk across to Bruce to plant a kiss on his lips.

'I can't believe it! We're getting married!' I exclaim as I go into the sitting room to find the telephone.

I call Sanda. She is a friend and also one of the registrars presiding over weddings and funerals on behalf of my Buddhist organization Soka Gakkai International, also known as SGI or SGI-UK. They have weddings once a month at our national centre, Taplow Court. The rest of the time, it hosts training courses for members from around the country. There is a spare date next year, but that would be too late for our purposes, as we want to be married before I'm pregnant. Sanda tells me that she'll look again and soon spots a space in four months' time – perfect. I swallow hard at the thought of how much there will be to arrange in just 16 weeks, but I'm a trained event producer, so I should be able to sort out our own wedding. I place my hand over the receiver to check the date with Bruce before confirming it with Sanda.

The booking complete, Sanda and I begin to chat. Our next challenge becomes apparent. Sanda is delighted with our news, but knowing that we've been happy living together for the past five years, she asks why we have decided to get married now, and in such a rush. Before replying, I check with Bruce that I can tell her about our disappointing circumstances.

Her response is characteristically supportive, but as I hang up I realize that this probably isn't the last time we'll be asked the same question.

'You know, once we start inviting people to the wedding, I bet you they'll assume that I'm pregnant or something; especially as I'm 39 and we've made no secret of wanting children.'

'Oh yes, you're right. I didn't even think about that,' says Bruce.

'How do you feel about telling people? I know our mothers have kept quiet, but they'll be feeling the pressure, keeping our secret from other members of the family. It's not really fair. They don't have anyone to support them at the moment.' Bruce's parents divorced some years ago, but both have new partners. Bruce and I decide to widen the circle of people we trust with our news yet again.

If we are lucky enough to have a child, everyone should know how much we are going to have to go through to get it. I hope they'll feel that they can support us when we need it. Over the next few hours we plan to tell everyone we can – full disclosure! I've had the frankly *brilliant* idea of piggy-backing the news of our difficulties onto an invitation to our nuptials: 'We have some good news and some bad news...' I don't know what reactions we're likely to get from each person, but at least we have the fallback position of talking about the wedding if there is an awkward silence.

In making up the guest list, we try to make sure that we don't miss anyone out – we don't want to be wondering whether we've told this person or that and risk forgetting when we next speak to them. We're confident that doing it this way, in one fell swoop, we'll be telling everyone we care about – if you are going to do a reveal, you might as well do it big style; get any embarrassment over in one go.

Telling our friends and family

We've decided to take advantage of the maximum number of witnesses allowed at our wedding. Marianne, my expert box-packer and constant support, was thrilled to be included, and delighted at the prospect of having a major role at a Buddhist ceremony – she's never even heard me chant before now. A second friend from my schooldays, Teresa, who lives some distance from London with her husband and two teenage children, has also agreed. We don't see each other as often as we would like, but nonetheless we remain close and always rekindle the same strong friendship, and giggles, no matter how long we've been apart.

Unable to choose between, and being inseparable from, his two oldest school friends, Bruce has decided on two best men: Matthew, a British Army major, and Ian, now a Big Shot in the city. Bruce, Matthew and Ian had many adventures together whilst at school and, if it were not for these two men suggesting the trip to France, Bruce would never have had an excuse to ask me out on a date. Having these four special people seated behind us will mean so much to both of us. We've asked Matthew to don his ceremonial army uniform for the occasion, plus sword, to add a touch more glamour.

With my newfound bravado, I make most of the calls inviting family, friends and work colleagues to our wedding and telling them about my infertility. As you might expect, there is a variety of reactions: 'Well mate, I'm sorry to hear that and of course, if you would like me to sleep with Caroline, I'd be delighted!' or, 'Shall I bottle some up and send it over? Two gallons enough?'

Some people want to know more about the whole situation – men who are not yet fathers suddenly being faced with the possibility that if it could happen to me, it could happen to them. My grandmother, who is 93, is amazing and wants to know everything, all the options for treatment. More than anything, she urges us to love each other and reminds me that loving each other is the truly important part of all of this.

Most surprising of all are the number of people who listen quietly and carefully, saying nothing at the time, but a day or two later take me discreetly to one side at work to tell me that they are in exactly the same situation but don't want anyone to know.

I discover a 'life lesson' in this short period of time: if you approach a subject such as infertility with absolute openness, honesty and candour, you will be amazed by the reactions. People gave me their heartfelt sympathy and respect and matched my honesty with their own.

The most difficult responses for me to deal with were from those people who didn't know what to say, or who were terrified of saying the wrong thing and so didn't say anything at all.

My oldest friend, Ian, was mortified by a misunderstanding between us when I thought that I'd told him about our wedding, asked him to be one of my best men and also told him about my infertility. He was in a queue at the bank at the time and had to hang up quickly when he reached the cashier. He called me back a couple of days later to apologize for cutting me off. During the course of our conversation, he told me all about a friend of his whose wife had just got pregnant and of how relieved they were because they had been trying for ages: 'Yeah, he's really happy 'cause he thought he might be a Jaffa. You know – no pips.' When I realized that he must not have heard the 'bad news' part of my previous phone call and explained my diagnosis once again, Ian apologized profusely. He says that he will think twice in future before making crass remarks to anyone else whose circumstances he doesn't know for sure.

6

Do we need another man in our lives?

A welcome break

I'm on my way to see Cathy, a fellow Buddhist. She and her husband, Mike, were amongst the first of our friends to make me realize that if Bruce and I wanted a baby, we should start trying sooner rather than later. She and Mike had tried to conceive for nearly four years, since she was 36 years old. Eventually she went to her doctor, who referred her to the local NHS hospital, where she was offered follicle tracking. She had daily scans, carried out mid-cycle, to track the growth of her follicles. The scans enabled her to predict more accurately the day she would ovulate. As I now know, there is only a small window of opportunity to get pregnant during each menstrual cycle. Cathy has just given birth to their baby boy, named Jack, at the age of 41.

Whilst chanting with her, the idea of using donor sperm weighed heavily on my mind. Now we're sitting around one corner of her kitchen table and Cathy is nursing her gorgeous son on her lap, listening attentively to my concerns. I tell her everything, explaining that Bruce is infertile. She stops me to ask, 'What does that mean? Does he have to change his lifestyle? Stop smoking? Reduce his stress levels? Wear looser pants?' she laughs, but then looks slightly embarrassed.

'No, not sub-fertile,' I correct her. Completely *in*-fertile – he has no sperm at all and never has had. He can never father our child.'

Cathy puts a comforting hand on my arm, cradling her baby with the other. 'So what will you do?' she asks.

'Well, we have to use donor sperm; we have no choice. My problem is that we've always fantasized about *our* child, of Saturday morning football in the spring and summer, running through leaves in the autumn, or tobogganing down the hill on trays in the snow. We watch other parents playing in the two adventure playgrounds with their kids. We were looking forward to being a part of all that...'

'Well you still can be, can't you?' she asks.

'What if I can't go through with using donor sperm? I'm still really uncomfortable with the idea. But if I can't, I deny Bruce his chance to be a father – I don't want to do that either.'

'What's making you hesitate?'

That's a fair question. Am I making too much of a fuss about all of this? I try to be honest about my feelings since the diagnosis.

'I know this sounds selfish and short-sighted, but no matter what happens now, I won't be able to have "the dream". I dreamt of conceiving *our* child, Bruce's child, not the child of a stranger.'

Cathy is still listening, letting me talk. I'm grateful; I trust her and feel safe to say more.

'I'm scared that I won't be able to love this child. Will I be able to love my baby enough if I don't see Bruce's features reflected back at me? I mean, if you'd had to use donor sperm, do you think it would have made a difference?'

Cathy pauses, strokes and kisses Jack's head, looks out into the garden for a moment and then back at me.

'I know that Jack looks like his father, so there's no question of whose child he is, but even if he didn't, he's *my boy*, you know? He's my boy whether his genes belong to my husband or not. I conceived him, carried him and gave birth to him. Besides, he'll so quickly become his own person, not someone forever connected to me or to Mike. I don't think it would matter to me how he got here. He's here and I love him.'

'The old nature/nurture question,' I say, looking up.

'If you like,' she replies.

Walking home past the playground in the park and the nursery school next door, I feel stronger than before. *I can do this. I want to do this – for me and for Bruce. It's all going to be fine.*

Checking for ovulation

I bought a Clearplan ovulation kit from the chemist shortly after our last clinic appointment. It looks exactly like a pregnancy testing kit. I've been peeing on the absorbent pad since day 11 of my cycle. I have to wait for up to three minutes to see whether a blue line appears in the control window, then watch for a second, darker, blue line to appear in the adjacent window. This darker line shows that the luteinizing hormone has reached a level at which it will stimulate the dominant follicle to bulge from the surface of the ovary, finally rupturing to release the egg. My ovulation isn't imminent if the line is not present, or is lighter than the control line. Today is day 17 of my cycle and I can see a dark, *dark* blue line, distinct from the other faint blue lines that have been appearing and disappearing over the past six days.

I can't help bouncing 'Tigger-style' into the bedroom to waken Bruce. I sit down on the edge of our bed, making my presence felt by nudging his body further towards the centre with my bottom. I peer into his un-bespectacled, vision-blurred eyes looking for reaction as I say: 'I'm working honey. I'm functioning – look!' Triumphantly, I hold up the testing stick.

'Umph! Spatial awareness honey, spatial awareness. What did you say?' He half sits up, screwing up his eyes, trying to focus on my face. Then he squints at the testing stick, but I lower it, realizing he can't see the magical blue line. Undeterred, I continue to babble.

'I've surged. I've been really worried all month that I'll miss it; I asked how I'd know if it was the surge. The clinic said "You'll know," and they were right. I looked this morning and thought: *that'll be a surge then.*'

'You're really excited aren't you?' says Bruce laughing, as I bounce up and down on the edge of the bed. He calms me down by grabbing my shoulders, preventing my next bounce. 'That's great sweetheart. So what now?'

'Well, this means that I'm ovulating, and *that means* that we can go ahead with a cycle.'

I hug Bruce and he kisses the top of my shoulder and the side of my neck. I offer to make a cooked breakfast, in honour of the good news; we should celebrate.

Cooking and eating our breakfast serve to distract me from clockwatching. I even manage to wait for a further ten minutes past opening because I don't want to seem over-excited. Inside I'm feeling childishly exuberant.

I book the scan and first set of blood tests for the following Tuesday, along with an appointment with my consultant, plus another with a nurse to choose donor characteristics.

Preparing for an IUI cycle

Today will be another meeting with another doctor – the 'head honcho' so to speak. I've been allocated a specialist called Mrs Storry.

She is exactly on time, floating gracefully towards us in a twin-set and pearls. Her hairstyle – a straight grey bob – gives her a somewhat severe appearance, but when she speaks, we feel welcomed and reassured. She asks us if we have any questions before she goes through my proposed treatment protocol.

'The blood tests will confirm your FSH levels and, as you are ovulating normally, we recommend a natural IUI cycle next month – it's less invasive and there's no reason why you shouldn't conceive naturally with the donor sperm. When would you like to begin treatment?'

'We've decided to get married.' I reach for Bruce's hand and he squeezes mine in response.

'May I offer my congratulations,' says Mrs Storry.

Bruce and I exchange a quick grin before I continue: 'So we'd prefer to delay any treatment until afterwards. I have to finish off a client contract first of all and by then we'll be only five weeks away from getting married, so we'd like to wait another three months. Will this affect my chances?'

'No, I shouldn't think so. FSH levels only change very slowly. As your levels are still well below ten, they are unlikely to change significantly in a matter of a few months. Would you like to proceed with the preparation for an insemination so that you can try a cycle as soon as possible after your wedding? Are you going on honeymoon?'

Bruce explains that he's working on a feature film, which means that we have to delay our honeymoon, giving us time to schedule my first insemination between the wedding and the holiday. I agree with Mrs Storry to use the next couple of months to put everything in place, ready to do my first IUI as soon as we're married. This also gives us time to save some extra money. We've decided to rent out our spare room to students enrolled for summer courses at our local language school. We have some cash, but we'll need more to pay for the wedding and the IUI, which will cost approximately £1000.

Mrs Storry brings our meeting to a close and sends us back to see Brenda for the next part of the process. We're pleased to see the same nurse who talked us through the first stage of this process.

Choosing donor characteristics

'Hello again,' says Brenda, stretching out her hand in greeting. We sit down expectantly.

'Now then,' she says, referring to my notes. 'You're having intra-uterine insemination. We'll monitor your natural cycle with regular ultrasound scans to assess the development of the follicles and your ovulation and, as there is no reason to suspect that you won't achieve a pregnancy on your own, we won't be using any ovulation-inducing drugs or ovary-stimulating hormones. It's better all round – medically and financially – and has much less impact on your daily life. It's less stressful to do this first of all.'

'Is the donor sperm – how can I put this?' *How embarrassing.* 'What does it look like?'

'Semen samples from the donor consist of two elements,' she replies, 'the sperm and the seminal fluid that makes up the ejaculate.' Brenda catches me sneaking a look of disgust at Bruce.

'Don't worry. We wash the sperm so none of the seminal fluid is inserted into your uterus. There are two reasons for this: as well as removing the risk of passing on any infections it may contain, the fluid can also be irritant to the uterus.'

'If the ejaculate fluid is an irritant, how do couples manage to get pregnant naturally?'

'Only sperm manage to get through the cervix into the uterus. But we do offer IVF treatment to couples who have problems with incompatibility. It eliminates the need for sperm to come into contact with vaginal fluids.'

'What tests do the donors go through?' Bruce asks, I guess to change the subject to something less biologically graphic. But it doesn't work.

'They're quite rigorous,' replies Brenda. 'You already know that we don't accept promiscuous men, and we also ask that the men we do accept refrain from intercourse for three days before donating.' She pauses before continuing: 'When we wash the sperm, any viral nasties such as HIV, hepatitis and other STIs that are held in the seminal fluid are removed. This is the safest way to use donor sperm.'

'So no buying fresh sperm over the Internet then?'

'It's a risk. That's why the HFEA is trying to ban the sale of fresh sperm through websites.'

Brenda explains that once we have chosen donor characteristics, the clinic select the closest match available from the frozen sperm in store. We all wait for me to ovulate, the clinic then thaws out the sperm and I come in for insemination.

I'm fighting the urge to run out of the room shouting 'No! No! I can't do it', but I manage to keep myself in check.

Brenda asks if we have any further questions, but we don't, so she pulls a piece of paper out of a draw in the desk and picks up a pen, scanning the first few lines of the form. She fills in my name at the top of the sheet then begins to tick boxes.

'Obviously you are Caucasian *(tick)*. We'll get your blood group and CMV positive or negative results from the lab. So we'll skip to the physical characteristics.' She leans forward and peers at Bruce's face: 'Blue eyes?'

'I've no idea,' replies Bruce.

'Well, green really,' I correct her. *Bruce's soft eyes melt my heart every time I look into them.*

Brenda's pen is hovering over the options for brown/blue/green on the page. 'Are you happy with blue or green?'

We look at each other, pause and then look back at Brenda and nod.

'Yes, I suppose so.' *This is so weird.* She keeps going.

'Brown hair? Medium skin colour?'

'Fair hair please, and fair to medium skin.' *I don't want to give up on the blond, curly-haired angels we've always talked about.*

'You know, the more selective you are, the harder it is to find a match. It's up to you of course...'

'I want to be happy with the selection offered to us.'

'Well, you'll only be offered one at a time.'

'Oh.' *Only one? This isn't what I imagined.* 'All the more reason to get it right, surely.'

'No problem. As I said, it's your choice.' Brenda smiles, then circles 'fair/brown' and 'fair/medium'. 'Height?' she asks.

'I'm about five foot eight,' Bruce replies, turning down the corners of his mouth in an upside-down smile of regret. 'Wish I was taller, but there you go.'

'Five eight or above?'

'Can we say five ten?' *I'm only five feet tall and always wished I were taller too; perhaps this is our chance to add a bit of height to our families. There has to be some benefit to this awful situation.*

'Build?'

'Medium to slim,' we reply. She marks the appropriate place on the paper.

'Nationality? Don't mind?'

'Any, as long as he's healthy.' *Is this nearly over? Please let it be over soon.*

'Education?'

I'm beginning to feel slightly uncomfortable – neither of us want to feel as if we're creating a 'designer baby'.

Bruce doesn't respond directly to Brenda's last question.

'What is it that we're meant to be doing here exactly? I mean, what are we trying to achieve?'

'It's such a bizarre process isn't it?' I comment, grateful for the halt in proceedings. Brenda nods and smiles gently as I continue: 'We're not trying to conjure up the child we've always imagined to be a combination of both our genes are we? We're trying to match Bruce's characteristics as closely as possible aren't we?'

Bruce and I haven't discussed what we wanted or expected prior to being in this room – how could we? It's so far outside our experience. This is really weird. We seem to be ordering up our child, a child that will definitely soon be a part of our lives, in the same way you place any order for delivery. It's exciting, I feel positive, but...

'Do you both have a further education?' We nod. 'If we are trying to match with you closely, then we should request the same level from the donor selection process.' She moves her pen to the section at the bottom of the page. 'Interests and hobbies?'

'Well I'm not sporty at all, but Bruce enjoys it.'

'Are your interests in the arts or more science based?'

'Both sides of both families do some of both,' I reply.

'I think I'll put "A good all-rounder!".' She laughs as she writes – underlining the exclamation mark. 'Right. That's it. All done. Is there anything else that you'd like to ask? When you call us to begin your cycle, we'll get you in to see the consultant for your blood results and so on.'

We don't ask any more questions because I'm a little overwhelmed by the whole process, and sense that Bruce feels the same. However, I remember to tell Brenda about our wedding plans. She congratulates us and makes a note on the file for October, continuing, 'Did I mention the legal limit of ten babies created per donor? Couples returning to have a second baby are sometimes disappointed to find no sperm is available from the original donor. This can be hard to accept, but it protects everyone, especially once donor anonymity is removed. More than ten offspring from one donor may be difficult to cope with, both psychologically and practically.'

'I think that makes sense,' Bruce replies.

I can't think beyond this first child, let alone contemplate going through all of this a second time.

'Now then,' says Brenda, closing the buff-coloured document folder, 'just the HSG to go, and you can begin treatment.'

'HSG?' *Not more prodding and poking. I can't believe how many hurdles there are to jump over before you get anywhere near an insemination. Couples who can conceive naturally have it so easy.*

'Yes, don't worry. It doesn't hurt. The proper term for it is a hysterosalpingogram.' I try to oust the image of a linguistically challenged, animated penguin from my mind. 'It's an X-ray procedure where the doctor injects a liquid up through your cervix and into the uterus. The passage of the dye can be seen on a screen and recorded on X-ray films.'

'A little like a barium meal?'

'Yes, that's right, but not taken orally of course. Have you had one of those?' she asks me.

'No, so I don't know why I said that really – it doesn't help me at all.' Typical. I'm just trying to sound blasé, or knowledgeable, or calm, whilst actually being ignorant, anxious and nervous. I laugh weakly and gesture to Brenda to continue.

'It will show us whether or not there are any blockages in the fallopian tubes. If there were, IUI would not work. It would be a waste of money because there would be a barrier to the egg and sperm being able to connect up and fertilize. We're aware of the financial implications of this treatment; we try not to put you under any additional unnecessary stress by carrying out futile procedures.'

Brenda logs our appointment for the HSG on the computer system and we leave the office, heading for the waiting room once more.

We stop chatting as the trendy Dr di Martino, who carried out my initial scan and clinical assessment, sweeps towards us with my notes under her arm. She is smiling warmly.

'Okay? We can go over to have an HSG now. I'm afraid that we have to use the hospital facilities over the road. We have no radiographers here, but there are only two of you today, so you shouldn't have to wait.'

Another lady, dressed casually in jeans and a red-and-white striped T-shirt, has joined us from the other side of the waiting room. We smile at each other for support.

'Are you nervous?' I ask her.

'A bit. I hope it doesn't hurt.'

We walk down the steps of the clinic, following the doctor, who is making polite enquiries about our holiday plans. But a tall, slim, fair-haired man walking towards me distracts me. I have to move aside to let him pass. He heads not towards the entrance to the clinic, but straight down to the basement where we've been told the sperm bank and cryolab are located. *Could he be a sperm donor? Will he be the father of my child?* I feel uneasy and look away quickly to focus on the taxicab on the road ahead of me.

Reaching the hospital, we're taken through to radiography, down a series of corridors, all grey and brown and in need of decorative care. There appear to be no staff around: 'It's just after lunch,' says the doctor, 'but still, I wonder where they all are?'

Her enquiry is answered by distant jubilant shouts of 'Goal!' echoing around and about us. Absorbed as we are in this all-consuming world of fertility treatment, the European Championship, and our country's progress in it, has lost priority for us. Two nurses make their way towards us, apologizing for the delay, but they are sure we understand…

The other woman is first to go through. Bruce and I sit in silence, both staring for the main part at the floor, occasionally looking up as muffled cheers or missed-goal frustration burst through the silence.

Twenty minutes later, it's my turn. Patient number one walks back through from radiography, looking bowed, but saying that it wasn't too bad. I'm still nervous.

In the examination room, one of the nurses helps me up onto the metal table, wraps a blood-pressure band onto my upper arm, presses down the Velcro fastening and begins to inflate it.

Dr di Martino is sitting on a low stool by my feet. I am asked to place myself in the becoming oh-too-familiar 'prone' position. *It's amazing how often I've had to assume the position of childbirth lately.* She comments on how calm I appear.

'Oh no she's *not*,' contradicts the nurse sitting by my head. 'Well not according to her blood pressure reading. Like a swan this one, aren't you my dear? All serene on the surface, but paddling wildly underneath.' She takes hold of my hand. 'It really isn't that bad, you know. We'll take care of you, won't we doctor?'

Dr di Martino nods her head, and tells me that if at any point I want her to stop so that I can take a rest, I only need to ask. This has the simultaneous effect of increasing my anxiety – is it so bad I'll *need* a break? – and making me feel less out of control and vulnerable.

The catheter and dye are passed through to my uterus without too much discomfort.

'Bruce and I are getting married, you know.'

'Congratulations. When's the big day?' asks Lisa, the doctor, without looking up.

'End of September. So I'm getting all this done, then I'll take a break until after the wedding.'

'Make sure you bring us the photographs won't you?'

'Of course. *Ouch!* Can you stop please?'

The cramping is sufficiently uncomfortable for me to want a break. I think I'm asking to stop simply because I don't want to feel completely passive any more. I feel so 'passed around' – not the clinic's fault; there's a lot to get through; I understand that. I soon reach the conclusion that the quicker I let the doctor get on with it, the quicker the discomfort will be over. I ask to carry on, so she shoots the dye through and withdraws the catheter.

'The results are good on the left – the dye shot out of the end of the fallopian tube – that one isn't blocked. But we didn't see any dye come out of the tube on the right. This means it could be blocked,' says the doctor. 'Would you like to see for yourself?'

Seeing the X-ray on the screen behind me is only possible by craning my neck backwards whilst trying not to move my legs, because they are still hanging over the end of the table. The doctor tells me that the tube could be damaged in some way. She advises me to wait for a follicle to appear on the left-hand side. This would give me the best chance of conceiving.

Apparently, the diagnosis on my right-hand tube is not 100 per cent conclusive. It's possible that the tube may just have gone into spasm as a reaction to the pressure of the dye – it may just have closed down in response to the invasion. I know how it feels.

Donor discussions

Bruce's work has taken him away for the week, so Mum has come to stay to keep me company and look after Barney while I'm at work. We've just settled down on opposite sofas to talk through wedding plans and have started to argue over the guest list, so much so that Mum changes the subject, asking me how the treatment's been going. I still have niggling doubts over whether or not I can deal with the donor sperm. I can't disguise my unease, and inevitably I confide in her, hoping for reassurance. Instead, she voices one of my secret fears.

'Have you thought that Bruce may not bond with the baby? If he can't and he leaves you, you're going to be in a mess.'

'*Mum!* We're only just about to get married. Don't talk about him leaving me already.'

'Well, darling, I'm only saying that if you're uncertain, it's best to tell him now so that you can both begin to come to terms with it.'

I know she's not being divisive and that her warning is coming from bitter experience. Her relationship with my father changed when I was born, as he distanced himself from the two of us, preferring to let her take full responsibility for my upbringing. It may have been a generational attitude, but all the same, she was left literally holding the baby. We both take a sip of tea at the same thoughtful moment.

'To be honest, Mum, it has crossed my mind,' I offer, looking down at the toes of my right foot as they scribe small circles on the carpet. I can feel my chest tightening as I hug my mug closer to me.

'If you're not sure darling, you need to say something,' Mum urges.

'I know that. I do try Mum, honestly. I keep asking him if this is really what he wants to do. He says that it is. If I say "No" at this point and he doesn't get to be a father, I'll always worry that he'll blame me later on and then he might leave me anyway. I don't want to be selfish, or give up before I've tried for him. If I can't go ahead, maybe I won't be enough for him in the future?'

'How do you know it's not the same for him? He might be encouraging you because he's scared that if he doesn't he'll lose you.'

We can't explore this any further, as I am crying again. Mum comes over to where I'm sitting to hold my hands in hers. I wipe my tears and clear my throat. She takes her empty mug and mine away towards the kitchen. I call her back from the doorway.

'Mum. You know, there's no sense talking about this now. I might as well get on with it.'

'Whatever you think is best, Caro,' she says.

'I'm sure it'll be fine, once the baby's born. It's what we both want isn't it? I'm so lucky to have a partner who is prepared to let me do this so that I can experience being pregnant and have a child who is genetically mine. I don't suppose there are many men who would agree to it. Yes, I'm *lucky* that he feels this way; lucky in so many ways. This is going to be fine.' I tail off, convinced, once again, that this will bring us even closer together, that I won't end up without the love of my Bruce.

★ ★ ★

Shortly after Mum returned to her home, I called Sanda, confiding my fear that no matter what I decide Bruce might leave me anyway. I asked her how we should begin to make these difficult decisions about our future and she offered one of the most valuable pieces of advice I received during the course of our treatment. She advised us to make each decision '100 per cent for yourself and 100 per cent for each other'. She explained that she believed this strategy would prevent resentment building up between us. My understanding of what she meant is this.

It's easy to fall into the trap of agreeing to take actions based upon your desire to make the person you love happy. But if you make decisions based on pleasing only your partner and not yourself, then you may come to resent the outcome. Similarly, if you make decisions based on selfish reasons, then you may put your relationship in jeopardy.

At this stage of our process, on one level I felt that I was taking a risk in going ahead with donor insemination, but I also felt that the risk of losing Bruce would be greater if I didn't. Bearing Sanda's advice in mind, I want to make sure that I have no long-term regrets – that I can't blame Bruce for not letting me try to become a mother and, at the same time, that he can't blame me for taking away his opportunity to become a father. If we are lucky enough to conceive, and with all the good causes we've made I'm sure that we will be, then all that matters is that we'll be parents. We'll have a family of our own and a child to raise and love. Our dreams will be reality at last.

7

Treasures of the heart

What a spectacular distraction from fertility treatment! I can't believe how much support we've had from our friends and family since we took the decision to share our secret with them. Our invitations have gone out, and as most of the 160 guests are not Buddhist, they don't know what to expect on the day; there's a real buzz of excitement around us. It's such a welcome antidote to the endless appointments, scans and tests. Even the nurses at the clinic have become involved, giving me their opinions on dress, flowers and catering options – I've been combining appointments with shopping trips in the West End to look at fabric, hats and shoes. We're nearly there and, looking back, nothing has been as perfect in my life for a long time.

The frock

I'm caught up in a flurry of female fuss and activity. Cathy has persuaded her mum to look after Jack for the day, so she is here with Penny, witness to my first phone call from Bruce, and Fiona, who now understands that no amount of lovemaking with Bruce is going to get me pregnant. Although Fiona and Cathy have never met Penny before, they have come together to accompany me around various department stores and bridal-wear retailers over the next week or two.

We're gathering strength for the task ahead in the fourth floor coffee house at Harvey Nichols, where Penny has arranged a personal shopper to guide me through the styles on offer.

'I've been looking for an excuse to do this for *ages*,' she remarks. 'My own day in a big frock seems further away than ever.' She tells Fiona and Cathy, 'I've just been promoted. It's a great job, but I'm always on the road, managing all our outlets. I never have the opportunity to meet anyone.'

This is a problem faced by many of my single thirty-something friends. Penny really wants children, but hasn't been in a relationship for some four years now and, at 37 last birthday, time is definitely slipping away. As I've been discovering the facts relevant to my own situation, she hasn't welcomed the knowledge that statistically her fertility is about to fall by 50 per cent. But at the same time, she and many of my other single girlfriends still have to pay the mortgage. That legendary glass ceiling seems to be showing no signs of shattering yet, so they can't let up on the career front in favour of starting a family before time runs out.

★ ★ ★

Five hours into our personal shopping experience and I'm exhausted. I've tried on everything from trophy-wife power suits to slinky, sexy frocks that wouldn't be out of place in a bordello. I've been laced, buttoned and hooked into bodices so tight that I can barely breathe; lifted into fairy-princess, meringue-netted skirts which made me giggle at the prospect of being able to smuggle half a dozen small children down the aisle underneath. Unfortunately, all the girls' efforts have come to nought. I have only learned what I don't like and what doesn't look good. And then there's my budget. We don't have much money to spend, as we didn't really plan to get hitched this year. I've tried to be happy in classic, clean lines, but it's not really me – my star sign is Leo and my taste is often quite flamboyant. It's a good job I'm marrying Bruce, with his love of elegant simplicity, otherwise we'd be living in the height of kitsch at home and the wedding decorations would be all feathers, fairy lights and heart-shaped balloons.

I received a call from Penny the day after our Harvey Nicks experience. She's put me in touch with a wedding dress designer called Christina who has offered to design and make an outfit to fit my budget. I can't believe she's doing this for me; I thought she'd be way out of my league on price.

At Christina's suggestion, we're meeting this lunchtime, in London's Berwick Street – home of a famous fruit and vegetable market, plus an array of specialist fabric merchants. This district is familiar to me because of my previous career in the theatre – it's a favourite haunt of costume designers and drag queens. I was often sent on errands here, buying props for the show stage management, collecting dry cleaning or swatches for wardrobe departments.

I've combined this trip into the city centre with an appointment earlier this morning at the clinic for more blood tests – the last ones before the insemination in October. Unfortunately, the nurses couldn't draw blood from my veins, so I have to go back this afternoon. This fabric-seeking expedition will serve as a welcome break whilst the crook of my elbow recovers.

Just as I look at my watch, wondering why there's no sign of my Frock Fashionista, my mobile begins to ring.

'Have you seen anything you like so far?' Christina asks.

'Nothing that I'm certain of. I like virtually everything I've seen, from cream georgette silk through burgundy and onto coffee-coloured chiffon with sequins. I'm incapable of making a decision. Please hurry! I desperately need your help.'

'You're hopeless,' she laughs. 'Don't worry; you'll know it when you see it. I'll meet you in the fabric bazaar next to the fake fur shop. See you in a little while.'

I press the disconnect button on my phone and move into the darkness of the shop behind me.

Christina seems confident that I'll recognize my dress fabric when I see it. What about my baby? Will I recognize my baby when I see it? Will I be as certain that I've done the right thing for Bruce and me?

Twenty minutes later, my new best friend and dress designer arrives, breathless and apologetic. She follows me over the threshold of an old-fashioned drapers shop, bursting with every type of cloth imaginable. As soon as we cross the threshold, I see the material for my bodice hanging seductively on the wall. It is azure-blue chiffon – brighter than turquoise – like a cloudless sky in high summer.

'There it is,' I say, pointing at it, waggling my index finger up and down.

'It's blue!' exclaims Christina. 'It's *exquisite.*'

The haberdasher lifts it down for us to examine more closely. The opulent detail reveals seed-pearl edging, shaped in scallops. Winding up and down its length are embroidered flowers with heart-shaped centres, finished with ruby-red or emerald-green beads. White thread petals edged with silver sit alongside acanthus pattern sewn in rich greens and silver and interspersed with more red, blue and green beading. The effect is stunning.

'It's an antique sari. It just came in today,' the assistant informs us. I'm in love with it, as I drape it around my shoulders, swirling gently by the main desk. Christina asks 'How much?' and I'm expecting to have to say farewell at this point, given the intricacy of the beading and variety of gem-like stones.

'Seventy pounds,' says the girl.

Christina looks at me incredulously: 'There are acres of fabric, Caroline.'

'Is there enough to make into a bodice?'

'Plenty.' Christina is nodding rigorously.

'We'll take it.' I hand it back to the assistant, who wraps it in tissue paper and folds it into a carrier bag.

Planning the ceremony

I completed and signed off my client contract yesterday and, as Bruce is working long hours six days a week on a film, we've decided that I won't look for another project until after we're married and I've had the first insemination. To keep the money coming in, I've let out our spare room as accommodation for foreign students, leaving the rest of my time free to sort out the invitations – which we're making ourselves – and discuss the order of service. A Buddhist friend, Oyin, is acting as liaison between Taplow Court, SGI-UK and the caterers. She works full-time for our organization and is well placed to keep everyone informed.

Our close friend, Sue, will be marrying us. She is licensed, within SGI-UK, as a lay celebrant, able to officiate the legal wedding contract as well as conducting the Buddhist ceremony. Our marriage is very special for her.

In the relatively early days of our relationship, I raised the issue of starting a family with Bruce. Perhaps it was a little soon, but I was already 34 years old and my biological clock was clanging ever louder in my body. Bruce dug his heels in, feeling unready and unwilling to take on the responsibility of being a father. We were not as adept at communicating as we are now, so I mistakenly assumed that his reluctance to have children meant that he wasn't committed to us. I began to withdraw from him, feeling that he would soon be on his way, looking for someone who was less desirous of a family.

I confided my plans to be single once more to Sue, during a summer stroll along the riverbank near her house in South London. She listened patiently as I listed my reasons, continuing to criticize Bruce's attitude to our relationship. When I'd stopped talking, she simply stood still, turned to me and said, 'Treasure him, won't you?' I could tell that she meant this with all her heart, and at that moment I realized that I was being extremely foolish: I had the potential to be really happy with my man. To avoid losing this potential for happiness, I had to change my attitude towards what we had together, and discover what was right about our relationship instead of only looking for what was less than perfect.

As I said goodbye to Sue at the train station, she stunned me by adding, 'I'm going to marry you two one day.' As she smiled and held both of my hands, she seemed absolutely certain that we should stay together. At the time, I didn't know what to say, but her faith and trust in us have helped us to see the best in each other over the years, and have shaped the care we take with each other every day.

A Buddhist ceremony consists of gongyo (reciting two extracts from the Lotus sutra plus four silent prayers) and daimoku (chanting the phrase *Nam Myoho Renge Kyo*). There's an optional ritual of sipping Japanese rice wine, known as sake, from three lacquer cups of increasing size, to symbolize the growing respect that we will develop for each other during our marriage. We've opted to include the ritual in our ceremony and have invited Bruce's youngest sister, Lucy, to be one of our sake 'maidens' and Heather, a theatre buddy of mine and constant companion on tour with *Aspects of Love* for nearly two years. She's been a fantastic support of late and it feels right to ask her to act as our second sake maiden. Both Lucy and Heather are also Buddhists, introduced to the faith by me.

Other than these few elements, we are at liberty to share with our guests anything within reason – usually readings, a poem or some music.

Sue, Bruce and I are all sitting around our dining table, thrashing out the details of our ceremony. Bruce suddenly jumps up: 'I know! Give me a minute. I wonder if I can find it?' He disappears upstairs. After a few moments, he re-appears holding a well-thumbed volume of poetry called *Love Poems* by Brian Patten and shows us a poem called 'A Blade of Grass'.

'I think it's lovely,' says Sue, as she finishes reading it. 'It's all about gratitude – very Buddhist.'

'It's perfect, honey. Where did you find it?' I ask.

'Oh, I don't know. I think we studied it at school. Until tonight, I'd forgotten all about it, to tell you the truth.'

Bruce and I have been into the park to pick a few stems of wild grass. This will be the image for the front of the invitations and order-of-service sheets. The delicate, golden ornamental grass stems fit with the theme of the poem and complement the simple, Japanese-influenced ceremony. The image is unpretentious and classy – very Bruce.

With help from a neighbour, Ray, who is a professional photographer, we produce an image of two of these grass stems, tied together in a love knot. The theme of the wedding is *One Love – it's now or never* and we've asked some of our professional musician pals to play the Ian Dury song of the same title on the day.

We have been granted special permission to bring Barney to Taplow Court as our Page Dog. I've sent off to a shop on the Internet for a doggie bow-tie and some spats for his paws. Sanda understands how much he means to us – he's been part of proving to us that having a family will be fun.

Preparing the reception

Three days to go. Mum and I have finally resolved our issues over the guest list. I'd forgotten that weddings are legendary for family squabbles and in hindsight I've realized how naïve I was to think that, out of consideration for the treatment we're undertaking, ours would be any different. To keep the peace, I have extended the number of guests invited back to our house for lunch and champagne, but we still have to work out how we're going to feed so many guests in our not-big-enough Edwardian terraced house and small courtyard garden. Oyin has taken over the management of the caterers as well as all liaison with the musicians – I have complete faith in her abilities. Janet, the wife of Bruce's good friend Ian, has taken on the task of decorating the garden and the reception area.

Mum and I have been shopping for hats and shoes. We've just returned from picking up my red feather headdress incorporating sections from the sari. It's wonderfully theatrical and, once the sari has been converted into a bodice and my cream georgette silk skirt is ready, will complete the Moulin Rouge look I've been aiming for.

The milliner's workshop is a long bus journey from our house, and when Mum and I finally get home and burst through the front gate, we're met with catering chaos. We approach our front door as Ray is leaving the house, sweating profusely and muttering, 'I only came round to drop off the photo for the invitations, but I was roped in.'

I rush past him into the hallway, through the kitchen, opening the door to the bathroom. But I can't get in because the sofa is propped up, leaning diagonally between the walls. The living room is full of 70 gold-backed chairs, stacked five high. The garden resembles a house clearance – filled with two armchairs, ten gate-leg rectangular tables and several crates of crockery.

'*Bru...uce!*' I shout up the stairs, from where I can hear more clattering and banging. Matthew and Ian are with him. I can hear playful insults coming from Ian and Bruce as Matthew tries his best to instil some military discipline and organization into the proceedings.

'Hi honey. Sorry about the sofa,' Bruce shouts back to me. 'It wouldn't go up the stairs.'

I can see that we're going to be thankful for our decision to book into a hotel the night before the wedding.

Bruce's best mates have been a real support to him over the past few weeks, especially Ian, who has thoroughly informed himself about azoospermia and what it really means to men like Bruce. He'll never make the mistake of calling anyone a 'Jaffa' again. Ian has confided to Bruce that he and Janet are now trying for a baby, so perhaps we'll all be pregnant together.

The hen night

I confess to just a hazy memory of my girls' night out, due to excess consumption of alcoholic beverages. Well, I'll soon be an abstemious paragon of virtue, an admirable wife and mother, won't I? Best make the most of it I thought...

All my friends contributed to my girls' night out: Penny organized everything, from the meal at my favourite local restaurant, to the waived entry fee into the nightclub. Marianne bought me a pink feather boa, Cathy a plastic tiara and L-plates, and Fiona provided a leopard-print sleeping mask with the word *Goddess* embroidered in bright orange on the front.

As I woke up – with a headache – the next morning, I remembered that my soon-to-be sister-in-law, Lucy, brought me home in one piece as promised. But apparently I embarrassed her and Marianne at the end of the evening by sobbing pitifully in front of a sign in the local kebab shop that said 'No chips on their own', while still sporting tiara and feather boa, because I didn't have enough cash to purchase a kebab as well.

The wedding eve

We're treating our witnesses to dinner at the five-star hotel where Bruce and I are staying overnight. Teresa, Marianne, Matthew and Ian, plus their respective partners, are all here, toasting our good health.

As the waiter takes our order for a bottle of champagne to toast tomorrow's nuptials, I'm taken aback by Teresa's request for tonic water.

'You teetotal these days?' I ask. But I know that she has been trying to have a third child, so can already guess the reason for her restraint. 'You're *pregnant* aren't you?' I whisper into her ear. She confirms that she's just nine weeks. As she's already suffered two miscarriages, I can't blame her for wanting to keep it quiet. I surreptitiously clink my glass against hers in covert congratulation.

'I'll chant for you and the baby. Here's to a trouble-free pregnancy – your good health.'

'Thanks, mate.' She nudges her shoulder against mine, and winks.

★ ★ ★

Amidst all the nitty-gritty of wedding plans, I have also become aware of the bigger picture, so to speak: the inescapable rituals by which we mark the passing of time and the passing of people into and out of life. Two weeks ago, Juliette, an elderly ex-colleague with whom I'd formed an out-of-work friendship, passed away from terminal cancer. Her funeral took place just 36 hours after her death, in keeping with her Jewish faith. As the end of her life was approaching, I was invited by her family to say goodbye to her in the hospice. Her great hero was Einstein, so I talked about the universe, the cosmos and my belief in eternal life whilst she held my hand, squeezing it gently from time to time, to let me know that she could hear me. She was unable to speak at this stage.

Taking a break from my frantic, activity-filled week to spend those last few moments with Juliette was a privilege. It was slightly awkward to begin with, as I'd never met her family before and didn't want to intrude on their grief. However, the awkwardness soon passed as they welcomed me, a visitor from their mother's long and valuable working life as an event photographer.

As if providing an antidote to Juliette's funeral, and a further portent of good things to come, being invited to a baby-naming ceremony just two days later lifted my mood, as well as further fuelling my reflections on the cycles of life. Roy and Angie, the proud parents, have also suffered the heartache of more than one miscarriage, which made their celebration even more special.

The contrast of experiencing these events so close together has made me truly appreciate the significance of my marriage to Bruce and its place in our own circle of life. This is just the beginning for us. By this time next year, we hope to be inviting guests to our own baby-naming ceremony. I'm already praying for trouble-free pregnancies, not only for Teresa and her husband and for us, but also for any couple fortunate enough to conceive.

The wedding morning

It was such a good idea to escape from the chaos at home and spend the night before the ceremony together. My hairdresser of 18 years turned up at seven o'clock this Sunday morning to pin my hair ornament in place and to dress my hair as a wedding gift. I'm just putting the finishing touches to my make-up.

Bruce keeps calling up to the room from his mobile asking me when I'm going to make my grand entrance into the hotel lobby to meet him. Matthew is in his army major's uniform, getting increasingly weary of being mistaken by tourists for a bellboy.

I feel like a queen as I make my way down the sweeping staircase and onto the arm of my soon-to-be husband. The look on his face and the love in his eyes tell me that this is going to be our perfect day.

The ceremony

We can hear the excited buzz of our family and friends as they take their seats, serenaded by Lucy, currently in her primary role as harpist, and our close friend Tim accompanying her on flute. They are relaxing the guests with a dreamy repertoire of Saint-Saens' *The Swan*, Caccini's *Ave Maria*, and Massenet's *Meditation from Thais.* Tim was delighted to be asked to play for our guests, his only proviso being 'I don't do Abba'. *We'll see about that,* we thought. Our Ian Dury tribute band and super-group are a mixture of non-Buddhist and Buddhist professionals, all friends from our theatre days. They are quietly standing by, just to the left of us onstage.

Proud parent Roy, whose baby-naming ceremony I attended last week, and who is also our Master of Ceremonies, welcomes our guests before giving the cue for our grand entrance. We are led by Sue and followed by our witnesses. As we glide towards the front of the hall, more than 100 friends are smiling at us and applauding – waves of goodwill and love. It's overwhelming. Whilst resisting the urge to hold up the procession by hugging everyone as we pass, we are delighting in our guests' surprise and puzzlement as the flute and harp change to *Take a chance on me*, by Abba. We can see people giggling as they get the joke. I sneak a knowing smile at Tim as we pass, and he narrows his eyes in mock disapproval, then winks, whilst still playing with absolute enthusiasm.

Bruce is whispering 'Enjoy it, sweetheart. I love you' in my ear as we walk up the three steps to the stage and take our seats.

Sue sounds the large, bowl-shaped bell and begins to chant. I hear Bruce, sitting beside me, chanting for the first time. I didn't ask or expect him to join in, but he's doing this for me, to show how much he loves me and feels a part of the ceremony. Cupped in his hands are the sandalwood prayer beads I bought him as a gift for this day. This sense of strong connection between us makes tears of joy roll down my cheeks.

The chanting continues for five more minutes, which gives me time to pull myself together. I turn around to Teresa, who hands me Matthew's militarily ironed linen handkerchief. Now comes the sake ceremony. The first hit of the sweet rice wine at the back of my throat calms my pounding heartbeat. Lucy is looking pretty foxy in her burgundy taffeta bodice and black leather trousers as she presents us, in turn, with each lacquered bowl. Heather, using all her musical theatre experience, is silently, but theatrically, presenting the red and gold teapot containing the sweet rice wine as if she were leading a solemn and momentous tea ceremony for the Japanese emperors. This, combined with trying not to giggle at the exaggerated faces of encouragement Lucy is pulling each time I take a sip, is making me smile.

I had breakfast more than five hours ago, and as I face the prospect of the third sip from the third and largest cup, I realize I'm beginning to feel fuzzy. I leave an extremely large helping for Bruce, who catches my eye, raising his eyebrows as I encourage him generously – all, of course, in silence.

The contracting words go without a hitch. This is the last time I shall repeat my maiden name. I'm taking Bruce's surname. From today, I will be known as Caroline Gallup. No one expected me to do this, as I have a well-established name and reputation in the entertainment industry. But it seems to me that if our child cannot be connected to Bruce genetically, at least we can feel more connected as a family by all having the same name.

All of a sudden we're declared husband and wife to an explosion of applause. We kiss each other, then Sue, hug our witnesses in turn, then step down towards the table where we sign the legal and Buddhist registers.

Graham, the unwitting cupid who brought us together at his production meeting all those years ago, now steps carefully onto the platform to read the poem by Brian Patten.

You ask for a poem.
I offer you a blade of grass.
You say it is not good enough.
You ask for a poem.

I say this blade of grass will do.
It has dressed itself in frost,
It is more immediate
Than any image of my making.

You say it is not a poem,
It is a blade of grass and grass
Is not quite good enough.
I offer you a blade of grass.

You are indignant.
You say it is too easy to offer grass.
It is absurd.
Anyone can offer a blade of grass.

You ask for a poem.
And so I write you a tragedy about
How a blade of grass
Becomes more and more difficult to offer,

And about how as you grow older
A blade of grass
Becomes more difficult to accept.

In Sue's wedding address she tells us about two mythical animals, representing the Buddhist view of marriage.

> 'The hiyoku is a bird with one body and two heads. Both of its mouths nourish the same body. Hiboku are fish with only one eye each, so the male and female remain together for life. A husband and wife should be like them.'[1]

She also quotes from the writings of the President of the SGI, Daisaku Ikeda.

> 'The husband is not the centre of the relationship, nor is the wife. It is not a question of who is the leader or who must make himself or herself a sacrifice for the other's success and happiness. Just like a song is a marriage of music and lyrics, husband and wife are equal individuals who, at the same time, perform a single melody of life together. What is important, I think, is how beautiful a song these two life partners can create together.'[2]

Sue reminds us to think back on these words from time to time, especially when difficulties arise to test our fundamental respect for each other. I look at Bruce, sitting on my right-hand side, hand splayed around his chin, elbow leaning on the back of his chair. *I love you, with all my heart. No matter how difficult this becomes, when I'm pregnant, when we're exhausted or worried about our baby, I'll always love you. We'll overcome any obstacles that life throws at us. Together I know that we're going to build the happiest of families.*

Who would have thought that the catalyst for this magical day would be a piece of legislation and a quirk of genetics? In the midst of everything uncertain, clinical and unpleasant, planning a wedding was something that had a guaranteed happy outcome. We had to do it for legal reasons – so that Bruce's name could go on the birth certificate – but emotionally it is so much more than that.

1 *The Writings of Nichiren Daishonin*, 1999
2 *A Piece of Mirror and Other Essays* by Daisaku Ikeda, 2004

8

The first insemination

Cycle one – day 10 scan

Time seems to have passed quickly and the crashing disappointment of Bruce returning to work the day after our wedding was soon swept away by the beginning of this process, as planned, four days later. Today is Sunday and I'm here for my day 10 scan, which should show the presence and progress of my follicles.

It's strangely quiet here in the clinic. I'm anticipating my first cycle of IUI with a mix of nervousness and excitement. We're missing the usual buzz of phones ringing and serious-faced clinicians or nurses in 'theatre greens' walking purposefully past us. In fact, there are no other patients here at all. The weekend receptionist asks us to take a seat. She phones through to the sonographer who walks towards us, hand outstretched, introducing herself as Bridie. This is our first meeting with her, as Dr di Martino carried out the last baseline scan.

We all go into the scanning suite together – I'm no longer embarrassed to have Bruce present. Bridie inserts the probe and begins scrutinizing my uterus lining and ovaries. The news appears to be good.

'There they are.' She sounds as if she really is pleased for me. 'You have three follicles, two on the right and one on the left. Do you see?'

I nod. 'Yes, that's good isn't it?'

'It looks like a strong cycle,' she replies.

She explains how the surge of LH triggers the release of the dominant follicle. The 'fingers' at the end of the fallopian tube capture it and the cilia – tiny hairs lining the tube – move it down towards the uterus. I have a concern.

'When I had my HSG, it was the right tube that they thought might be blocked. If that's where the follicle is released, what happens?'

'Well, if it is blocked and your dominant follicle is on the right-hand side, the sperm and egg wouldn't be able to meet. The nurse will advise you in a moment, but you may have to cancel the cycle. Let's hope not.'

Bridie sees me glance at Bruce, then back at her as my mind has raced on to the question of finance.

'This cycle has already cost a thousand pounds. What about the payment we've made?'

'Oh, don't worry. If that's the case, then I'm pretty sure you would get a refund or a credit to use on the next cycle. But don't let's assume the worst just now. Wait and see what the nurse tells you. I'll see you in a couple of days for another scan.'

She leaves me to get dressed. Bruce holds the door open for me as we take the couple of paces across the corridor to the nurses' room, where we are greeted by yet another new nurse, who tells me her name is Jameela.

I'm disappointed not to see Brenda or Clodagh – it's all feeling a little like a conveyor belt, albeit a comfortably carpeted one.

The nurse is studying three biro crosses marked on a chart printed on pink paper and stapled into my notes. The crosses rise on the scale as they go from left to right across the page, charting the growth of last month's dominant follicle.

'Well, this looks good Caroline. Please begin testing your urine from tomorrow, and come back for a second scan when you've had your surge. We have a donor for you, would you like some details?'

'Oh yes please,' I say, beckoning Bruce to squeeze into the tiny room with us.

Jameela tells us the donor selected against our criteria is British; he's an accountant. He has brown eyes, he's five feet eight inches tall, and is of medium build. His interests are listed as reading and travelling. Bruce frowns and leans against the doorjamb. I feel my heart sink. Both Bruce and I have artists and scientists in our families, and all Bruce's relatives are tall and slim. I definitely wanted someone with fair hair so that we stood a chance of creating a child close to a mix of Bruce and me. I feel no connection with this donor.

But it's only his sperm we're talking about here; I don't have to go on a date with the guy. I can't believe how prejudiced I'm being. It's just...perhaps I'm feeling disloyal to Bruce? Oh, I'm being ridiculous.

I force myself to focus again on what Jameela is saying. I'm sure I can rationalize and overcome my disappointment, at home, in private. I should make sure that nothing stands in the way of our rapid progress through this process.

'Are you still happy to test your urine at home?' asks the nurse. 'Is that okay?'

I clear my throat. 'Yes, yes, I'm sorry. Yes. I'm absolutely fine with that.'

Cycle one, day 11 – first test for hormone surge

According to yesterday's scan, there are follicles developing on both sides. Even if the dominant follicle grows on the side that might be blocked, I'm going to go ahead with the insemination. I can't stand to wait another month, and they did say that the tube might just have gone into spasm when I had the HSG. My blood test results were all fine; I hadn't ever had Chlamydia, thank goodness. I'm excited about this; really optimistic.

A new brief to work on

I've decided to accept a short contract of work. I'm needed for just nine days, to project manage a charity event for some regular clients, starting the day after tomorrow. The fee is welcome, and as the work follows on from the end of a previous project, it doesn't carry the extra stress of taking on a new brief for unfamiliar clients. Taking into account the timing of the cycle, the contract will be over well before any potential insemination days.

My first client briefing session didn't get off to a very good start when I had a telephone conversation with the head of the trustees for the charity about my availability and the hours we would allocate to the project.

'It depends on the hours you need and when,' I said. 'I may need to be more flexible this time and restrict my hours at weekends.'

During my last contract, I had been able to work evenings and weekends as necessary and was prepared to work long hours to get the job done. His curiosity was therefore aroused by my apparent reluctance to be as freely available. I'd just come back from the clinic and I suppose he caught me off-guard, because I explained that Bruce and I were having fertility tests, possibly leading to treatment, which would mean I needed flexibility and time for appointments. First of all he tried to sympathize by telling me that his wife was also having problems. I could tell from his tone that he had made the usual assumption that the problems lay with me. I decided, foolishly as it turns out, to correct him and educate him about the existence of azoospermia. I had hoped that he would just wish us well and mind his own business. But instead, obviously not listening to my explanation, he interrupted me mid-sentence, his voice flushed with pride, with a blindingly insensitive statement which clear took my breath away: 'I, on the other hand, have the opposite problem – I've been told that I could populate the *whole of Europe* with my sperm count.' My heart sank.

As I will encounter time and time again, on hearing about an otherwise healthy member of their gender *not* being able to father children, something is triggered in certain men that seems to compel them to make sure you know that they don't have that problem. They give testament to their virility to the point of absurdity.

I ignored his vulgar remark and wished him every success with their efforts to conceive in the future, asking him to extend my best wishes to his wife.

Instead of signing off gracefully, he couldn't resist another go, proving to me that he hasn't listened properly to my explanation of our particular problem: 'Well, nice talking to you. I'm sure we can accommodate your treatment requirements. And don't worry, even if you have no luck for a while – at least it'll be fun practising.'

I was speechless as I slowly pushed the button disconnecting our call.

Cycle one, day 12 – rejecting the donor

I'm depressed about the accountant. I've tried to joke about it with Bruce by saying that we can't accept him as our donor because we're both rubbish at maths – how will we help with homework? Each time I chant about it, I begin to cry or feel depressed. I know it's only sperm, but it doesn't feel right.

Bruce is home from work. He walks through the front door, removes his jacket and places the empty cup from his morning coffee on the kitchen counter. I say that I need to talk as he sits down next to me on the sofa.

'I keep crying when I think about the donor. I just don't want this one: an accountant of medium build with brown hair. I don't want to be rude and

I know that I should be grateful that we have a chance, but the pen sketch sounds nothing like you. Am I being stupid?' I'm looking at Bruce for permission to say 'No' and ask for another donor.

'No, I don't think that you're being stupid, or ungrateful. We are supposed to be matched with someone who looks physically similar to me, so that we stand a chance of having a baby that looks like a mix of the two of us. Remember, those letters from the Donor Conception Network said that we have to be ready from the moment our child is born for those "Who does he or she look like?" questions. So, if you're not happy, say "No" and ask for another donor.'

I'm so relieved. I feel as if a benevolent breeze has blown a dark cloud away from me.

'I'll call in the morning then.'

Cycle one, day 14

Everything is in place now, except one major element – the clinic hasn't yet found us another donor. I call them every day to see if there's any news, but no luck so far.

I've nearly completed the nine-day contract, but juggling work with appointments and scans has proved tricky. The clinic told us that they have women 'dropping in' during their lunch hours. I don't see how, as the last scan appointment is just before lunch and as I have no control over my cycle, I can predict which day I need an appointment with the clinic. So far, I've had to take time out during working hours and make up for it during the evening. If I were my client, I might think twice about sending through any more work. Am I good value for money? But what does that say about my attitude to women struggling with young families or those in exactly my situation?

At least once I'm pregnant my clients will perhaps be more sympathetic and familiar with my need for time-out for various antenatal check-ups and maternity leave. Of course, I can't claim maternity payments because I'm self-employed, so I'll just have to keep working as long as possible.

★ ★ ★

I've just switched on my mobile and it's ringing. I recognize the number – it's the clinic.

Jameela confirms that they have another donor to offer me: 'He's a French medical doctor with proven fertility, which means that he already has a family of his own. He's five feet ten inches tall, with blond hair. He has an athletic build; likes reading, creative writing and sailing; he's…'

'That sounds great,' I interrupt. 'Yes please. He sounds fine. I'm happy with him.'

I'm feeling quite giddy. I can almost see this handsome doctor, sailing with his family on a bright sunny day in Cannes or Nice or maybe even Le Touquet, where Bruce and I flew kites on our first date. Our donor is sitting in the stern of the boat, manning the rudder; his attractive wife and two blond children are swapping from side to side of the vessel as they tack along the coast.

Coming from scientific genes will fit in well with our families: if our child shows any propensity for medicine, I can always say that the genes *could* have come from the donor, but it's also in the family, so it could be from my father, who was a general practitioner, or Bruce's mother – that would also help our parents to feel connected to their grandchild. It's a shame that my father isn't alive to meet his grandson.

Jameela's voice snaps me out of my fantasy: 'Good. Well I'll change the donor code on your notes and call the cryolab so that they can prepare the sperm. We'll see you in a couple of days then.'

Cycle one, day 17 – surge and final scan

It's day 17 and I had my surge of LH this morning. I rang the clinic immediately and they were able to fit me in for a scan. The follicles are a good size, at 17 millimetres. Apparently, the optimum range is between 17 and 21. So it's donor insemination day in two days' time – Saturday.

Cycle one, day 18 – first insemination day!

Yet *another* new nurse introduces herself, and I'm afraid I instantly forget her name. She apologizes: they're not quite ready for us. She asks us to take seats in the waiting room. I had hoped that Brenda, or even Jameela, would be doing this, but I suppose that nursing rotas can't be co-ordinated with the cycles of individual patients as nothing in IUI is exactly predictable.

The waiting area is less plush than downstairs. It's more spacious, but has blue, hard-plastic stackable chairs. There are three doors leading to consulting room number three, the laboratory and a treatment room. Bruce opens his book and begins to read. I grab a magazine from the table in front of us. We wait to be called.

After about 15 minutes, a man and a woman emerge from the treatment room. She is wearing jeans and a red jumper and is clutching her handbag and coat in front of her stomach. She smiles at me, a little too weakly for my liking. *It must hurt.* Her partner grins broadly as he places his hand gently on her back, ushering her towards the stairs as they say goodbye to the nurse, who turns her attention to us.

'We'll just be a few minutes. Sorry you've had a bit of a wait.' She turns and walks back into the treatment room, closing the door behind her.

★ ★ ★

I feel depressed as we enter the insemination room, but if I look around objectively at the brightly lit space containing a treatment couch, sink and floral privacy curtain, it's not too bad. It smells clean, but not antiseptic, and despite the fluorescent tube, there are also sidelights on the wall to soften the surroundings. I think it's the sight of the two metal leg rests attached to the end of the couch and the Anglepoise lamp facing me from between them which makes my stomach somersault. This is not going to be easy, or remotely romantic.

I haul myself onto the couch once I'm stripped from the waist down. A second nurse covers my knees with a blanket. 'What's your name?' I ask her.

'Anita,' she replies, smiling.

The first nurse, who had disappeared into a side room, now returns holding a test tube containing a fluorescent pink liquid. I resist placing my ankles inside the metal, semi-circular supports and remain with my knees pulled tightly up to my chest while she explains the procedure.

'Here's the sperm,' she says, jiggling the tube in front of my face.

'There's not much there,' I comment. 'I expected more liquid. And it's *pink*!'

'Well, there are thousands and thousands of sperm in there, maybe millions, and it only takes one,' she says. 'We keep them in this pink-liquid medium once they have been washed. You know that there's no seminal fluid around them don't you?'

'Yes, yes. Actually the colour makes it easier to accept.' I'm beginning to feel a little happier. *This is just sperm. Just sperm, no other man involved. My man is here with me, and always will be.*

Anita then gives the instruction I've been hoping to delay for as long as possible: 'Okay then. Can you rest your knees on the metal supports please?'

I put my hand out to my right, where Bruce is sitting. He takes it into his and gives it a squeeze. I turn away from the nurses and towards Bruce, as the lamp is angled to get a good view of my cervix. The catheter is unwrapped from its sterile packaging by the nurse whom my wayward mind has unhelpfully called 'The Sperminator' in place of the name I can't remember.

Bruce gazes into my eyes. I see that he is completely in love with me. This *must* be the right thing to be doing. I'm looking back at him trying to replicate that 'look of love', but it's almost impossible to turn my mouth up at the corners to fake a smile. I hope I'm not letting him down. I hope he can't tell that, for me, this experience is proving clinical and uncomfortable.

This whole thing seems a bit odd. By doing this, somehow we're going to end up with a baby. Does not compute. This is happening to Caro; I just happen to be here. If I wasn't, it could still happen. Thank goodness that liquid looks nothing like sperm.

I feel undignified and slightly embarrassed that Bruce is here with me. As they warned me it might, my groin is cramping, trying to reject the plastic tubing being pushed past my cervix and into my uterus. I want it to be over. I make myself numb. I switch off my emotions, but want Bruce still to know how much I love him, so try to keep smiling. After about five long minutes, 'The Sperminator' withdraws the catheter. It stings slightly as it slides out. Anita stands up, straightens her apron and pats me on the top of my foot: 'You can take your legs down now, it's all over.'

I move my ankles from the metal supports and sit up, carefully straightening my legs down onto the treatment couch.

'Okay then. Well done,' says The Sperminator. 'Please do a pregnancy test in 14 days' time. Let us know the result either way.'

I feel embarrassed that I can't remember this woman's name. And that I can't get Arnold Schwarzenegger's voice out of my head.

'Arnie' continues: 'You'll be four weeks pregnant if the test is positive. Even though it'll be only two weeks since the insemination, your GP will take your week-count from the first day of your last period.'

'Is there anything I should or shouldn't do during these two weeks?'

'Well, you should assume that you are pregnant, so no alcohol, and no excessive exercise. Don't go mountain climbing or parachuting if you haven't done it before.'

'I've heard that you shouldn't drink caffeine.'

'There's no real evidence to suggest that caffeine does any harm to the baby in the first few weeks. Most women are behaving completely normally for the first weeks of pregnancy; they usually don't do a test until they are six weeks pregnant. It's up to you, but it's "precious cargo" you're carrying isn't it?'

I touch my stomach instinctively. 'Should I stay lying down or anything; or stay here for a while?'

'There's no need,' she says with a smile. 'The sperm can't fall out.'

The nurses both leave the room, wishing us good luck. I carefully slide off the couch and begin to get dressed. Even though I know that I can't lose any of the precious sperm, I'm moving more mindfully than usual.

'How was that?' Bruce asks.

'Pretty awful to be honest.' *It felt as if I was there to have a PAP smear, only my lover was present – very strange.*

'At least we were looking into each other's eyes,' he says, helping me with my coat.

'Yes,' I reply flatly, trying to think of something positive to hide the fact that I felt nothing at all. 'I'm glad you were with me.' I feel a tear pricking at my eyelid, but manage to blink it away, and gather myself up. 'Come on, let's get out of here.'

We're trying to imbue this procedure with some sort of meaning, some sort of emotion, but I don't really feel anything. My mum has been encouraging me to make sure that we are close tonight, that we make love and make the day something special. I can't say I feel particularly gushy or romantic.

We walk down the steps outside the clinic. Having paid for the cycle at the start, this is one of the few occasions that we don't have to go to Accounts before we leave.

'Are we in a hurry to get home honey, or shall we have a look around the shops?' We're still holding hands and I'm feeling much more upbeat now that it's over.

'Yes, if you like. Are you feeling up to it? We'll do whatever you want.'

Bruce puts his arm around my waist, pulls me closer to him and kisses my cheek. We cross the busy main road and enter the covered market to find a stall selling baked potatoes. After a stroll around the nearby shops, another cup of coffee for Bruce, and herbal tea for me, we make our way back home to snuggle up on the sofa together.

Reality bites

I'm in bed before Bruce, who is brushing his teeth next door in our half-decorated bathroom. For the moment we will have to postpone all the plans to re-style our new home: the bathroom needs updating, the house needs a new roof, new windows, fitted wardrobes, a new kitchen – all of that will have to wait. The cost of the treatment must come first. I don't mind. At least we'll have our own baby, and when it's born we won't care how it got here, how it came into being; we'll just love him or her with all of our hearts.

Bruce enters our bedroom, turning off the main light as he passes. Reclining luxuriantly, I joke: 'So, do you think I'm pregnant yet?' *I must be pregnant mustn't I? How can the sperm not meet my egg? Surely there's no way they can't fertilize: where else can they go?*

He smiles: 'It's strange isn't it, to think how much our lives are going to change if you are? We could be *parents* honey. You and me. *Parents.* Nothing's ever going to be the same again.'

I'm sure Bruce won't mind that I don't really feel much like making love as we'd planned. I expected to feel excited and sexy, but instead I feel detached, a bit unfeminine. We can have a close hug instead. I need to feel his arms around me, to feel loved and cared for.

Bruce turns away from me to switch off his bedside light. I expect him to turn back towards me and open his arms for a hug, but he remains lying on his side, his back to me, and simply says 'Goodnight, honey', blowing me a kiss over his shoulder.

I feel a sudden stabbing pain in my chest. I think I know what this means, but it can't be true, can it? I have to ask for what I need: 'Can I have a cuddle please?'

He sighs, and after a pause says, 'I don't really feel like it. Sorry. I need to go to sleep.'

My chin starts to tremble. 'I need a cuddle. Please hold me. I thought we said that we were going to make love tonight, and be close, and make it special?'

He reaches out and turns his light back on. He turns the top half of his body towards me, but looks out into the middle of the room. 'I'm sorry. I thought I could cope with this, but I can't. I can't seem to bring myself to touch you.'

'But I might be pregnant! What are you saying? Are you saying that you've changed your mind about me doing this?'

'I thought I could cope, but now I don't think I can deal with the reality of you having another man's sperm inside you. I'm sorry.'

'Well it's a bit bloody late to change your mind. *You* were the one who wanted this to happen. What the hell do I do now?'

'I don't know, honey, I don't know. I didn't know that I was going to feel like this.'

I feel detached from Caroline. We've done our best to make this romantic, but it hasn't worked. When we left the clinic, we went for lunch and for a walk along the riverbank, but it felt like we were filling time. I wanted to be actively doing something, but from what the nurse was saying, things have changed: Caro must be careful, behave as if she's pregnant. It's such a false situation.

I know that I've hurt Caroline by rejecting her advances; she obviously wants to make love as planned, but I can't.

I throw back the duvet and sit on the edge of the bed with my head in my hands. *What am I going to do? I have to get out of the bedroom and be on my own. I need to get away from him, to cry or scream.* When I speak, my voice is small, calm and quiet, the complete opposite of the maelstrom I feel inside.

'I'm going downstairs to make a cup of tea. We'll talk in the morning no doubt.'

I grip the countertop in the kitchen as I wait for the kettle to boil. I could do with a brandy, but the nurse said not to do anything I might regret, so I'd better stick to tea instead.

I turn on the television, but mute the sound, and stare at the flickering adverts as I nurse my cup, sitting alone in the dark. I'm numb.

After a while I feel the calm on the outside unite with a calm spreading on the inside and I begin to feel sleepy. I climb the stairs and sit on the edge of the bed, trying not to wake Bruce, who is now snoring peacefully, still facing away from me. I carefully get into bed, positioning myself as far away from him as possible, not wanting to risk contact with his skin for fear that he'll pull away from me once more.

Cycle one, day 19 – day one of the two-week wait

The sensation of having live sperm from a man I've never met swimming around inside me is strange, because there *is* no sensation. But I do feel different. I keep wondering if a sperm has met one of my eggs and pierced the outer membrane, managed to get through to fertilize it. Sitting by the window in the conservatory, I can hear Bruce in the kitchen. I know we have to talk, and Bruce has offered to make our coffee. He's waiting for the kettle to boil, but he's silent. Normally we'd be chatting by now.

I'm still angry and hurt and don't know what to say, but Bruce is as courageous as ever as he breaks the silence.

'I'm so sorry about last night. I don't really know what to say, but we probably need to talk…'

That afternoon we talked until no more talking would help. The only consolation we found was in our conclusion about the totally alien nature of the procedure: there's no comparison with natural conception because making love is pleasurable. Nature has it sussed – she gives you something to enjoy in and of the moment, quite apart from the procreation that may or may not be occurring.

Now all we can do is wait 14 days for the result.

9

Trials and traumas

I still can't feel anything happening in my abdomen, so I've decided to go onto the Internet to find out what should be going on at this stage of the fertilization process. It'll give me something to think about as the days slowly pass. I've been called for jury service for the whole of next week, so at least I'll have a distraction – take my mind off the second week of waiting.

I notice that I am stroking my belly as I read about ovulation and fertilization. I'm trying to keep the egg warm, encouraging it to move along on its journey to my womb. In the first three days, some time between yesterday and tomorrow, the sperm will be trying to pass through the cumulus cells that surround the egg like little clouds. Then our intrepid sperm has to bind to the shell surrounding the egg. *Shell? So, I'm not a girl, I'm a chicken.* The head of the sperm then releases some digestive chemicals to create a hole in the shell, which allows the sperm into the egg. But the journey isn't over yet. The sperm has only reached the antechamber of the egg – talk about playing hard to get. Only one sperm will fuse with the shell of the egg, and both the shell and membrane have mechanisms to prevent additional sperm from entering.

The knight in shining armour ***does*** *exist – and every pregnant woman has enacted her own intra-corporeal tale of chivalry even before she pees on the little white tester stick.*

After our crusading sperm has found his way through the maze into the fairytale castle and brought down the portcullis, the head of the sperm dissolves – *that seems a bit harsh* – allowing the chromosomes from the egg and sperm to merge and the process of cell division to begin. The fertilized egg, or *zygote,* floats down the fallopian tube until about day six, when it reaches the uterine lining. All being well, it will implant and continue growing into an embryo and ultimately a foetus.

Insemination day plus 5

I have pains in my stomach and I feel sick. Maybe it's a good sign. I wish I had X-ray vision to see what's going on inside.

Insemination day plus 8 – jury service begins

I'm due at Crown Court by nine o'clock – it's only ten past eight and I'm about 20 minutes away. I've left plenty to time to get there so I don't have to rush. As I approach the imposing entrance, I feel a little intimidated.

'Good morning. Where do I report for jury service please?' I ask the man guarding the barrier.

'Straight through Madam,' he says, pointing to a revolving door leading to a large marble-clad lobby. 'Report to the desk on the right and they'll tell you where to go.'

Insemination day plus 9

I'm so bored. Bored, irritated and restless. I thought that I wouldn't have time to count the days until I can do the pregnancy test, but I haven't been called to hear a case yet. I'm counting the *hours*. After a training film, signing in and completing a questionnaire, we sit around in a vast room with uncomfortable seating, low tables and old magazines – it's not dissimilar to a large-scale version of all the waiting rooms we've been in lately. The only difference is that I don't have Bruce to talk to. All I can think about is whether I'm going to be a mother by this time next year. I wish I had someone to confide in, to share my anxiety. I can't phone out of the building, I'm on my own at lunchtime; I can't go home and I can't settle to a book.

Insemination day plus 10

The stress of waiting for this pregnancy test seems to be taking a toll on me. Today I experienced what I now assume to have been a panic attack.

I had some time to kill during lunch-break for the courts, so I decided to visit the *Britain at War* exhibition just down the street from London Bridge Station. I walked up to the authentic 1940s ticket booth and paid for a ticket. The ticket office attendant pointed towards an entrance inside an elevator – the exhibition is built underground. It's a mock-up experience of the Blitz in London – 'set piece' family sitting rooms with crystal set transmitters, dance halls, makeshift sleeping bunks in an underground station, and pubs complete with darts and bar billiards. The layout is a one-way-only tour; no way back until you reach the exit.

The final scene is a representation of a night of bombing. At the top of a ramp towards the end of the bar is a double door with a notice saying, 'Please take a moment to allow your eyes to adjust to the dark before moving forward.'

I pushed the door only to see pitch-blackness in the next room and hear the sound effects of bombs falling and screaming. My face prickled, my stomach knotted and my legs seized up. I tried to move, but I couldn't. I pushed the door again, but jerked away from the swing-back. Out of nowhere, a fear of death overwhelmed me and I began to shake uncontrollably. I had to wait until another visitor appeared to ask for help. An elderly lady and her husband walked through to the exit with me, holding my arm and reassuring me, guiding me until I reached street-level once more. I've never experienced anything like it before, and I hope I never will again.

Insemination day plus 12

To my horror, I started to bleed today – just spotting, but it's definitely blood. I have to wait until lunch break at the courts to call the clinic. I find a relatively private alleyway by the river, between two office buildings. They answer quickly, as usual: 'Good afternoon, how can I help?'

'Hello. Can I speak to one of the nurses please? It's Caroline Gallup.'

Brenda picks up and I explain that I have started to bleed, two days early, and ask what to do regarding the scheduled pregnancy test. Her advice surprises me.

'Bleeding is often a sign of the fertilized egg implanting in the womb – it displaces some of the lining whilst it's burrowing into position to develop. You should do the pregnancy test anyway, regardless of the bleeding.'

'So, I could still be pregnant?'

'Yes, absolutely.'

I hang up, making my way back into the afternoon court sessions with a renewed spring in my step. I call Bruce.

'So what's the verdict? he asks. 'Has it been 12 good sperm and true?'

'Very funny,' I reply. 'It only takes one, as you know full well, but the news is good as a matter of fact – I still might be pregnant.'

That evening, Bruce insists that I rest up on the sofa while he cooks our favourite meal. He is taking such good care of me these days, I have nearly been able to forget the hurt I felt the night he rejected me two weeks ago.

Pregnancy test

I feel numb as I look down at the testing stick. Not pregnant. I call the clinic to tell them that the insemination has not worked.

If I try to look on the bright side of all of this, I can at least say that I have one treatment cycle 'under my belt'. Now I begin counting towards the next cycle. This is 'day one'. That's all. Not a failure, just another 'day one'. I'm relieved as well that Bruce and I have more time to talk about how he feels, faced with the reality of donor sperm inside me, and about whether or not we should try again in a hurry.

Healing time – our belated honeymoon

We've finally managed to fit in a few days away, which we are treating as our long overdue honeymoon. We have talked about the fact that we missed the boat by not taking a honeymoon straight after our wedding. We thought it would be okay, but it wasn't, it definitely wasn't.

We are booked into a luxury country house hotel for just four days – the only days Bruce has free in his ramped-up work schedule. It doesn't disappoint. On hearing about our nuptials six weeks ago, the management have upgraded us to a suite of rooms in the old coach house, and invited us to dine, for our first evening meal, in the private salon, with a complementary bottle of champagne thrown in.

★ ★ ★

I'm lying next to Bruce in bed watching a weepy movie – my emotions have travelled well beyond the celluloid story, opening the emotional pathway into the disappointment of my failed insemination. I've started crying and can't seem to stop. Strangely, it feels good – a release. Bruce is holding my hand as I reach for another tissue.

'Is this helping?' he asks. 'Shall we watch a different film, or are you feeling better for a good cry?'

'I think so. I don't know. I'm sorry,' I sniffle.

Reflecting on the disastrous night of the insemination, I still can't explain why I closed down. I'm not one for analysing my feelings in depth. I think on quite a small scale and wasn't thinking big as I lay in bed that night. I just think about what I'm feeling in the moment. That night, I just felt like I wanted to be closed up. I didn't feel like being very big and extrovert. I felt like being very introvert. I could see that my reaction was hurting Caro, but I also knew that whilst I never intentionally wanted to do that, I felt an even stronger urge that I didn't want to make love and I wasn't going to be bullied into it. It would have made me feel worse. It's unfortunate that she hadn't told me that all she wanted was a cuddle; I thought we were still following the plan we'd made earlier.

★ ★ ★

Bruce wanted to spend the day reading by the indoor pool. He seems to want to be alone. We still haven't talked about the failure of the first insemination, or Bruce's rejection of me. Even when we had the perfect opportunity amidst my tears last night, we both pulled back and focused on the movie instead. There seems to be nothing we can say at the moment to make it better. Perhaps it's too big for us to look at – I'm assuming that we both prefer to leave well alone for a while. To give us more space, I'm going horse riding this afternoon – taking advantage of the local amenities.

★ ★ ★

Trotting up and down hills on bridleways through still-leafy woodland and past farm buildings and meadows, I appreciate the tranquillity. The only sound is the rhythmic creaking of the leather saddle beneath me. My guide rides ahead of me, making small-talk. I can reply without any soul-searching, only talking about our wedding, where we live, what we do.

I'm glad in one sense that the insemination didn't work. At least if we can have some fun together now – celebrate our marriage – it might make the next time more bearable. But, according to my consultant, we can't relax for too long. We must try again soon, whilst I'm still less than 40 years of age. All these years waiting for the right moment to start a family, and now it's a race against time.

Time alone to recover

I'm booked onto a Buddhist study course at our European centre. These are bi-annual opportunities to spend time with my fellow Buddhists, to study the philosophy in more depth, and to refresh my faith and practice. Although we've only just come back from honeymoon, Bruce understands that this time away performs a different function in my life. I am going with his blessing, just for five days, whilst he starts work on another film. My mum will be keeping him company and looking after Barney whilst I'm in France.

As a special treat, my erstwhile wedding planner, Oyin, and I are staying over in Nice the day before we drive to the centre, sightseeing in Marseille and along the Cote d'Azur. After a delicious evening meal, we retire to our shared room, in preparation for tomorrow's journey. I fall asleep as soon as my head hits the pillow.

★ ★ ★

How did I get here? Am I awake? I screw my eyes tight closed, then open them again and try to focus in the dark. I am curled up, naked and freezing, on the wrong side of the locked closed bedroom door, slowly starting to panic as the creeping cold of the stone floor registers on my bare skin. A marble-tiled staircase stretches away in front of me, in two directions, up to another floor and down to reception.

I've been sleepwalking. What can I do? I'm cold. 'Of course,...Oyin!' Turning around, I begin to knock on the bedroom door to waken Oyin. I knock quietly at first, not wanting to risk alerting other guests. I can't even imagine the horror of trying to explain my predicament to a stranger. It would be horribly embarrassing in my native language, let alone in my schoolgirl French. *I wish Bruce were here.*

No response. I thump harder. Nothing. Panic. I'm really cold now.

What are my options? I could go down in the lift to reception, but what then? 'Excusez moi, mes vetements, ils sont disparu! Non, je ne suis pas une lunatic, je suis...' No, I can't, I'll be arrested.

I have to try to find something to wrap around my body. I stand up cautiously and climb the stairs in front of me. I stay bent over as I tiptoe up the steps onto the landing above, gingerly checking around the corner for any wandering guests. *How on earth did this happen?*

On the upper landing I find a laundry hopper. I eagerly look inside, but to my utter disappointment it contains only two pillows without pillowcases – no bed linen. The pillows will have to do. They're better than nothing, and at least I'll have something to sit on outside the door, and something to cover my front. I resume a slow, methodical thumping on the door. *I'll just have to keep going until Oyin wakes up.*

After about what seems like an age, my roommate opens the door, frowning in her sleep. I scuttle straight past her, leaving the door to swing shut, and dive into my bed to thaw out. Oyin remains silent, sliding straight back into her bed before falling back to sleep. I pull on the nightdress that I had discarded earlier due to the heat in the bedroom, pulling the covers tightly around my neck and shoulders.

★ ★ ★

The drive from Nice to Trets is easing my tension, and Oyin and I are still laughing about last night.

'I can't believe that you were locked out, or that I didn't wake up as I was letting you back in,' she says, shaking her head from side to side.

We try to take in as many of the sights as possible prior to paying the toll and driving onto the A8 in the direction of Aix-en-Provence.

The entrance to our European centre stands on a hill, close to a medieval market town, about one hour's journey from Marseille. It comprises a large, modern meeting hall, a smaller lecture and chanting hall, accommodation block and canteen. Pine forests, yew trees, laurel plantations and spectacular mountain scenery surround the buildings. European members of SGI come here for up to five days to study, chant and meet other members. Courses always invigorate and uplift me, and I think of this place as more of a spiritual gym than the retreat associated with other types of Buddhism. Here, I feel safe to be really honest with myself. This time I'm determined to see what to do next, and how and when to do it. Despite our lack of success, I feel that my baby is still out there, floating amongst the stars, just waiting for the right set of circumstances to be in place so that he or she can burst into life. I believe that the baby we will eventually conceive will have chosen

Bruce and me to be its parents; the donor is just the means by which he or she is able to come into our lives.

I'm sure that I've overcome my queasy feeling about using donor sperm, but still have some unidentifiable misgivings. I bump into Oyin, walking back to the accommodation block after supper. We find a quiet spot away from the main accommodation block and sit on a low wall together in the evening sun as I share with her my growing unease about doing another cycle so soon. She knows that Bruce and I had some problems with the last insemination, and of course she pointed out to me that my sleepwalking incident in Nice was likely to be stress induced.

'It's not that I don't want children and I do want to try again; I just feel rushed. The doctors keep saying that I can't leave it too long; that I don't have time on my side...'

'Who says that you don't have much time?' she asks.

'The doctors. What do you mean?'

'Well, think about it. If you want to leave it for six months, then do so. Your body won't lose the ability to have children overnight, or even over the course of a few months for that matter. I'm sure that the doctors are advising you that you don't have *years* to waste, but six months isn't going to make any difference is it? Check with them of course, to make sure, but if you really feel under pressure, that's not going to increase your chances of success either.'

I breathe a sigh of relief. *Of course* she's right. I've become caught up in the panic of medical speculation, based on the best advice that they can give me. But less time doesn't mean *no* time. I just have to calm down, and take things at a pace I can cope with. If I want to chant about this for a month or two, to get my head around it all, and relax, at the same time giving myself the best possible chance to succeed, then I can.

Delaying our next cycle

I've summarized my conversation with Oyin for Bruce and asked him for his opinion.

'If you want to take a break before the next treatment, that's fine,' he says. 'Don't rush into anything you're not happy with.'

'Don't you mind? Are you sure?'

'No, honestly. When are you thinking of delaying until?'

'The New Year? How does that sound? It'll give us a chance to recover financially as well.'

And so we agree that I'll call the clinic in the morning and say that I'm taking a break for Christmas. I'll try again in January – I'm sure that I'll feel better about all of this by then. Perhaps the New Year will bring us more luck. What's more, I can enjoy the Christmas party season without feeling that I've sacrificed myself on the altar of the goddess of fertility.

10

Footprints in the sand

'Something doesn't seem right,' says Bruce's sister. After her starring role in our wedding, Lucy is back at home in Australia, where she emigrated a couple of years ago. We stay in close touch and are in the midst of one of our mid-morning catch-up phone calls.

'What do you mean "doesn't seem right"?' I am surprised by her lack of support and a little taken aback, as this is the only negative response we've had from any member of our respective families. I've just explained how difficult it was for me to cope with the first insemination, but that I feel okay about it now and that we have decided to try again in the New Year. I expected more enthusiasm from someone as young and dynamic as Lucy.

I am unnerved by her reaction and realize that she may well be reflecting my own fears back to me. I still feel unsettled: perhaps we are defying Nature by forcing this baby into existence. Maybe we're meant to be childless.

I ask her to define what she means by 'not right'.

'My problem is that something in your tone of voice makes me feel that you're still unconvinced that you want to do it again. I think it's a massive step to take if you're not sure Caroline. *I'm* trying to imagine how I'd feel carrying a stranger's child if I loved someone else.'

I interrupt her, instantly angered by her seeming lack of support. 'By having a donor child Lucy, we have the chance to have a child that is genetically related to me, I get the chance to experience pregnancy and birth, and Bruce will be a dad from the outset, and be a part of bringing a new life into the world.'

Overhearing my end of the conversation from the conservatory, Bruce has walked into the room and is extending his hand, indicating for me to pass the phone over to him. I tell Lucy that I'm going to pass her on to her brother.

'Hello, Sis. How are you? Settling back into Life Down Under? …No, we're both happy to carry on, I mean, we've hardly given it a good try yet…' Bruce pauses. By the face he pulls, I guess that Lucy is still not convinced, but I'm quite surprised by the strength of what he says next.

'Look, I know that you're trying to think deeply about what we are doing because you care about us and want to understand, but to be honest, whether anyone in the family approves or disapproves, this is not a family decision. Ultimately, it's up to us to take whichever course of action makes us happy. After all, it's going to be our child. He or she will be raised and loved by us, to the best of our ability. All we can do is take all the help and advice that's on offer from the professionals and make our decisions accordingly.' Silence. 'I don't know whether that helps at all, or whether it all sounds a bit harsh. Do you want to speak to Caro again? Okay. Well, 'bye for now. Take care. I'm passing you back…'

He puts a questioning 'thumbs-up' in my direction and I nod in approval to what he's said as I take back the receiver.

'Hi there. Is that any better?'

'At the end of the day,' she says, 'it's not going to be a democracy vote on what you guys decide to do is it? Strangely enough, I can totally accept that,' she laughs. 'This whole idea is so outside my realm of experience, but I don't want to feel weird about it. If you guys keep going with this, I want to feel that I can support you sincerely. I think I'm going to find out more about it from this end – inform myself.'

The donor anonymity laws changed in Australia some years ago, so I suggest contacting the Australian equivalent of our Donor Support Network: the Donor Conception Support Group of Australia.

What makes a family?

Bruce's grandmother has requested a visit so that she can see our wedding video. She's 94, nearly blind and wants to watch the replay of events on her big-screen television. She also wants to celebrate our union and has created a 'bridal suite' for us in her guest bedroom. We love Nana.

Bruce's grandfather, who originally trained as a cabinet-maker, moved the family from the South East of England to the West Country, taking advantage of post-Second World War farming grants. Approaching their cottage-style farmhouse is like going back in time: over one hour's drive from the end of any major roads, it is very isolated, flanked by high, dense hedgerows. Nana's faithful cattle-dog – a thick-coated Border Collie – is stationed by the front door, barking to alert his mistress to our arrival.

We walk through the kitchen, across the foot-worn flagstones and into the front parlour. Sitting around the vast, deep inglenook fireplace, drinking tea from the best china cups, Nana is in reflective mood.

'I keep wondering you know, what footprints I've left in the sand,' she says. There's a note of concern, or sadness, in her voice.

'What do you mean Nana?' asks Bruce.

'It's a poem by Longfellow I think.' She quotes the lines on her mind:

Lives of great men all remind us
We can make our lives sublime
And departing, leave behind us
Footprints on the sands of time.

(Henry Wadsworth Longfellow, 1807–1882, *Resignation*)

'I wonder what footprints I will leave.'

'What do you mean?' I ask. 'You've had children and have ten grandchildren.'

'Have I loved all my family enough?' Nana continues, as if she hasn't heard me.

Bruce jumps in: 'Surely you're not being serious, Nana? You're the kindest and most loving person I know. You've cared for all of us, encouraged us and supported us. You've loved us. We can feel it. *No one* could have done more than you. I have such happy memories of being down here on the farm.'

Nana seems reassured and asks us how the treatment is going. We say it hasn't worked this time, but we're not giving up hope.

'Beth has had her fair share of heartache you know,' she says, referring to one of Bruce's cousins. 'They tried for a baby for many years, but it never worked. Of course, you know that they eventually adopted Reece and then, two years later, little Annie. I love my adopted grandchildren just as much as if they were my own flesh and blood.'

Nana fondly relates the story of how Beth's first adopted son reassured his newly adopted sister about the court procedure to legalize their status as members of their new family: 'He was only five, but he said to his two-year-old sister: "Oh, it's nothing to worry about. You go into the courtroom, the nice judge is sitting at a big table; he gives you a chocolate and a fluffy dinosaur toy, then asks you whether you'd like to carry on living in your new place. You say 'Yes', then he stamps a piece of paper and you have a new mummy and daddy – it's easy!"'

We all laugh at the delightful simplicity of his view.

★ ★ ★

During the long drive back to London, Bruce and I talk about our visit. We discovered an unexpected link between Nana and myself during this trip: she was born and brought up in my hometown, a very small market town on the borders of Herefordshire and Monmouthshire. She moved away in the mid-1930s, whereas I moved in, as an 18-month-old baby, in 1964. I even knew the exact house where Nana used to live, just one road away from my own. It gives me a tangible sense of connection with Bruce's family.

'It's not until you think about all the members of our family that you realize how many different people we love as our own,' says Bruce. 'When you think about it, our extended family comprises adopted children, step-children, children born into same-sex relationships, but all of them are embraced and loved without prejudice or exclusion. If we ever had any worries about how our donor child would be viewed, I think this visit has definitely put those fears to bed, don't you?'

'Definitely,' I reply. 'There's no doubt in my mind that not only are we doing what feels right for us, but we'll also find support and love from our family.'

'I didn't mention this at the time, but Mum made me promise that when our child or children are old enough we will send them down to her for the summer holidays. I couldn't believe it, but she's kept all the toys and play equipment from the nursery group she used to run, specially for her future grandchildren.'

'No wonder she never parks the car in her garage,' I laugh. 'It must be chock-full of stuff.'

Bruce and I feel on top of the world – we're as clear as we've ever been that what we are doing is right for us. Now all I need is a low-stress, flexible job that allows me to attend appointments at the clinic while still bringing in some cash to help with all the extra costs of treatment.

11

Good omens and then...

I received a call today asking me if I would like to provide temporary cover for an administrator at my Buddhist headquarters, Taplow Court. My chanting for good fortune has evidently worked, as I can't think of a better environment to be in at the moment – my spiritual sanctuary. Succour and financial support all provided in one fell swoop. The hours are flexible and I start just after Christmas.

I'm trying not to hope for too much good fortune all at once, but I think my chanting could have worked in another area as well – my period is late. Could it be that I may not need that second insemination after all? I won't tell Bruce just yet, as I don't want to build his hopes up until I've done a pregnancy test.

Christmas Day

I had no need to raise Bruce's hopes about becoming the natural father of our child; my own dreams fell away with the arrival of my period this morning, which is much later than usual, even taking into consideration the erratic length of my cycles. I had no business hoping that his diagnosis was untrue. How stupid of me, and what an unwelcome Christmas present. Bruce keeps asking me what's wrong, but I don't want to admit my foolishness, especially as he doesn't share my faith. I'm going to keep quiet, call the clinic to book a second cycle and get on with what we have to do.

Cycle two, day 1

It's a new year and a fresh cycle. I took a deep breath and rang the clinic to book in for a day 9 scan. I'm chanting for a baby very strongly now – maybe three babies, or four! Why limit ourselves?

Cycle two, day 9 scan

I can't stop crying, as I have only one tiny follicle on the left – the side that isn't blocked – but a larger one on the right. This means that the one likely to 'pop' when I ovulate is on the wrong side *again.* When I saw the nurse, she warned me that this cycle may not be a strong one – those words sound all too familiar – and said that I need to be prepared to cancel the treatment for this month. Next month both the follicles may be larger and of better quality and perhaps on the right – the *correct* – side as well. It seems a lot to ask for; we could be waiting for months for all the factors to be right. I can't believe how contrary my body is being. There must be a way to connect my emotional desire and my physical body. Sometimes I can keep a cold away if I don't have time to be ill, so perhaps I force my body to work with me, not against me, with my willpower. I'm going to use the strength of my desire and the power of my faith to make the follicle on the right diminish and turn the one on the unblocked side into the dominant one.

Perhaps when I chant I should focus on how much I love Bruce and try to visualize us as parents – maybe that will be enough to bring our child into being. This morning, at Taplow, I met Oyin in the staff kitchen, making herself a cup of coffee. She asked me how I was getting on.

'I still wonder if we're doing the right thing, to be honest. I seem to be seeing a lot of signs that my body is not with me on this one,' I admit to her.

'You know, I'm sure this baby wants you and Bruce as its parents. There *is* no relationship with the donor, only with the two of you. However your baby gets here, you are Mum and Dad and always will be. Whatever grows inside you will be a blessing. Please try not to worry about right or wrong; just do what feels right and keep chanting for the best and happiest outcome for both of you.'

★ ★ ★

Despite my determination to remain hopeful and confident, I often find myself bursting into tears unexpectedly. I think I've worked out what all the crying is about – I'm grieving for the genetic child that Bruce and I will never have. Our donor-conceived child seems different from the boy I saw in my fantasy. Perhaps I am not getting pregnant because I was still attached to that other child. Perhaps I am blocking the arrival of our donor baby.

How dreadful if my strong will, stubbornness and resistance to the process have cost us time and money. I only hope that I've done enough to make this insemination successful, to give us a real family, not an imaginary one.

Cycle two, day 12, second scan

I did it! I have two, 12-millimetre follicles on the left and *none* on the right. The follicles are small, but I'm not discouraged; at least they are on the left at last. This means that we can go ahead with the cycle.

I had another call from Lucy this morning. She contacted the Donor Conception Support Group of Australia and had a long chat with one of their volunteers. She's signed me up to receive their newsletter and sent off for a book called *Let the Offspring Speak*. It's a transcription of the speakers, most of whom are donor-conceived children, at a conference held in 1997 following the removal of donor anonymity over there. It will be like a look into the future for us.

I'm feeling really positive. I've been asked to come back for a final scan on Tuesday. I should be having my surge around then.

Cycle two, day 15, third scan

I've had no surge as yet. I'm going to the clinic on my own for the scan, as Bruce has to work today. I'm feeling buoyant as I take the steps two at a time and push the front door of the clinic. I know the routine now: I announce my arrival to reception, then pick up a scan form and begin filling in my details. The clinic has a system whereby you fill in a short form and circle whether you are there for a scan or a blood test. I then slide the form into a Perspex pouch attached to the nurses' station door and wait to be seen.

The sonographer, Bridie, soon appears, walking behind her previous patient. She collects my form from the pouch, smiles, looks up and walks towards me.

'Hello, Caroline my dear. Please come through.'

I jump up out of my seat, walking briskly with her into the darkened room, and begin to get ready for the scan.

'How are we today then?' Bridie asks cheerily to distract me as she positions the probe to find my uterus lining.

'I'm feeling good thank you. At least the follicles have seen sense and grown on the correct side this month. Very well behaved.'

'Absolutely.'

'Now I just hope that they're growing nicely.' I relax and wait for news.

Bridie is having trouble finding one of my ovaries: 'The tricky wee thing. It's slid around the back. Come back won't you?'

I didn't know that they could be 'tricky', or that they moved around. I ask Bridie to explain.

'Oh yes. They don't stay in one place. If you think about it, your body is soft and malleable; in diagrams, of course, everything is facing you and static, but in reality the fallopian tubes are cylindrical and floating around attached to one side or the other of the uterus... Ah yes, I've found it.'

She is staring at the monitor screen as the blue, grainy picture on the screen reveals a tiny, black, dent-like circle. No matter how many times I look at this picture, I'm still not quite able to discern all the parts of my anatomy as clearly as Bridie's trained eye.

'This is the left ovary and there's your follicle. I'll just do the measurements.' She moves the cursor to one side of the follicle, clicks the mouse and leaves the image of a white cross on the screen. She then moves the cursor to the other end of the follicle, clicks again and a cross appears, together with a measurement, in the top left corner of the screen.

'Okay?' I ask. Bridie is quietly surveying my notes from the last scan. She doesn't look at me, but still at the screen, moving the probe around gently. When she answers me, it isn't good news.

'It hasn't grown at all I'm afraid. It's still only 12 millimetres. You may have to abandon this cycle. Let's have a look on the other side, just in case...'

There's nothing we can do. There are no other follicles on the right-hand side. This was good news on Tuesday and now it's a disaster. My heart sinks. Bridie is not trying to be falsely optimistic, instead she commiserates. Once she has recorded the measurements on my chart, removed the probe and placed it back in the holster at the side of the machine, she goes to cleanse her hands whilst I get dressed. She talks softly to me as she follows me out of the scanning suite, her hand on my shoulder.

'That's bad luck, Caroline. I'm sorry. But see what Brenda has to say; you never know, all may not be lost this month.'

But it is. Brenda advises me to cancel. She shows me this month's chart as compared to the insemination I had in October last year. At the same point, my follicle was more than 14 millimetres and growing at a much faster rate – the optimum size is somewhere between 17 and 21 millimetres at this stage. There doesn't even seem to be any point in discussing this with Bruce. I say nothing, but Brenda needs a decision.

'It's up to you, but this really doesn't look like a good cycle. I would advise you to abandon this month, and wait. We can refund the remaining money, or put it towards your next cycle...'

'I see.' I can't take this in. I can't bear the thought of making this decision and having to walk out of the clinic. *I thought my determination had turned this situation around.* Brenda waits, pen poised above my notes, and I can see no alternative. 'You'd better cancel it then,' I say. My nurse nods and closes the buff folder; I notice that she stopped short of putting a biro line through the crosses on the pink chart, or writing any notes. I appreciate the sensitivity.

As I walk home alone, it's cold and getting dark. Bruce won't be back for at least four hours. I decide not to call him at work, but to go home and chant.

★ ★ ★

The underground is packed. Squashed in amongst the throng is a mother with a baby in a pushchair. Despite the crush created by bodies in close proximity, the child is protected within her own pushchair space, managing to reach her pink woollen-clad foot to chew on the satin ankle ribbon threaded through the bootie. The look of pure, concentrated joy on her face is attracting the attention of the passengers surrounding her, causing them to squash closer together, creating space enough for everyone, including me, to watch her, along with her loving mother. She has the wrapt attention of most of the carriage as we all 'Coo' and 'Aaahh' at her antics.

★ ★ ★

I reach our front door, turn my key and step inside our home. Barney greets me with less enthusiasm than usual. I've noticed that he is slightly more distant and 'head-shy' with me these days. He goes to Bruce now for cuddles and comfort. I know why; it's obvious to me. It's because these days I cry all the time and animals don't like their owners to be upset. Around me he feels insecure. When Bruce comes home from work, Barney sits across

Bruce's legs at the first opportunity: man and dog on the floor by the fire, or on the sofa, watching telly. From this safe place, our dog seems to view me with what looks to me like disappointment or dismay. It's as if he sees right inside me. You can't hide your true feelings from an animal.

I catch hold of Barney's tail, allowing it to slide through my hand as he walks away from me towards the cupboard containing his treats.

'Would you like a treat, sweetheart?' I follow him, reaching up into the cupboard – the least I can do is make my homecomings associated with something lovely for him, even if he mistrusts my mood. He settles on his blanket and I watch him contentedly and noisily chewing his treat. I decide to go upstairs to chant for a while – to work out how to break the bad news to Bruce.

My chanting room, called a butsuma, is set up in the smallest bedroom at the back of the house. There's a simple sofa bed, plus the cupboard, or butsudan, containing the scroll I focus on when I chant. The butsudan is lavender blue (a personal choice) coated with ten coats of lacquer applied over the course of many weeks by its maker. The lacquer gives it a sumptuous appearance, disguising the more practical, economically considered MDF base material. It sits on top of a small, Chinese-style low sideboard, bought from the local antiques market.

As I sit down in my low wicker chair and cross my ankles, picking up my prayer beads and placing my hands together, fingertips touching, I begin to recite the mantra out loud: *Nam myoho renge kyo, nam myoho renge kyo, nam myoho renge kyo.*

I expect, as usual, to feel first reassured, then strengthened and focused, and to gain a feeling of courage permeating my thoughts, leading to a certainty of the actions I should take to see positive changes in my life. But today is different. Instead of clarifying, my thoughts freefall into chaos.

My faith isn't working. That's why my body isn't co-operating. I'm not good enough; I don't want this child enough. I'm trying to make it happen but it isn't working. Everything I've believed in for the past 11 years is rubbish, it's pointless, worthless and ***doesn't work****.*

I lose track of time, beating myself up mentally and bombarding myself with my perceived inadequacies. By the time I hear Bruce's keys in the front door, I'm sobbing fit to burst. He hears me from the hallway.

'What's the *matter* honey? What's *happened*? What is it?' As he's racing up the stairs, I am coming out of the room to meet him at the top. He reaches out to touch me, but I brush past him and head down towards the kitchen. *How can I tell him how desperate I feel, how useless I've been?*

'We want different things, Bruce,' I sob, walking past him. 'I *hate* this. I don't want children any more. I don't want to do this any more, I *can't* do it any more.'

Where are all these words coming from? Do I really mean what I'm saying? Is this the truth I've been trying to get to?

'Would you love me even if I don't do this? I know that you say that you gave me enough time to make a decision about whether or not I was okay with this, but I know that it was really a case of "you take as much time as you like, but make sure you come to the *right* decision". You sit there like the bloody Buddha,' I shout at him, 'telling me you've come to terms with your diagnosis. Well that's fine for you; *your* life isn't the one that's changed – *mine* has! You just get to go to work as normal in the morning and come home at night. It's fine for you.' I'm screaming at Bruce, but it feels like a release. *I love Bruce, but I can't seem to stop saying these awful things to him. What's wrong with me?*

My lovely, gentle husband is just standing in front of me looking hurt and mystified. *Why doesn't he come and hug me, hold me?* I feel empty. My arms hang at my sides like dead weights as I carry on sobbing. He's saying nothing, although I can see that he wants to. I can't wait any longer for him to reach out. I run down to the bottom of the stairs and on into the kitchen. I don't look back to see if he's following me. My world has reduced down to my body and a six-inch air space around it. Nothing can get past this barrier.

I rush through the garden and into the office – to do what, I haven't figured out – I lean against the doorframe for support. My legs feel weak; I'm looking out into the kitchen but all the images are blurred. I close my eyes and feel hot, wet tears run down my face again. My eyes are sore, red raw; I want to stop crying but the sobs just keep coming. Bruce has followed me, but my outburst seems to have paralysed him. He stands in front of me asking me what on earth is the matter, but I can't stop sobbing.

I drop to the floor, curling into a tight, tight ball once I hit the wooden planking. The floor sinks away from me, becoming a deep, black hole into which I'm falling and spinning. The blackness is a blanket, enfolding me in comfort and warmth, calming me and damping out the pain. I feel hollow; my organs and bones disappear, dissolve, until just my skin is left – wrapping paper, but no present inside. I want to die; I want to feel nothing. I want this thing I *can't* do to go away, to stop pulling me on into perhaps more pain and an uncertain future with a child who will not be Bruce's, no matter what we do. If I could only block out the process, sleepwalk through the clinic, the couches, the scans; wake up pregnant and onto the next phase where I can be a normal part of society, not being ricocheted around the edge of the mothers' circle. I want to be a part of the mothers' union. I want to sleep, to be rocked, and be held – by my mother, by Bruce, by me. My tears engulf me. I am wailing, keening, I can't breathe – I'm breathing out, but I don't want to breathe in again.

Slowly and quietly crawling out of the depths of my despair, I become faintly aware of a small voice in my head telling me, 'You still have a choice.' I feel myself choosing to stop crying. I make a decision *not* to sink further down or lose control any more. I can choose to go on. I am not entirely powerless.

★ ★ ★

It's over and done. I'm calm. I still lie curled tight, unable and unwilling to move. I'm finished. Dead to everything I thought I was. I no longer have the energy to be angry. I submit to whatever is to come, but I don't want to lose control. I *can* choose what I want to do next.

'Caro? Caro? Please tell me what's wrong.'

It's Bruce, kneeling down beside me on the floor in the narrow doorway. His hand is hovering above my shoulder.

'It's okay. Please…hold…me.' I can't cry any more. I have no more tears. 'I feel as if I want to die. But I don't; I just don't know what to do any more.'

'Why are you so upset? What happened at the clinic? I should have come with you.'

'I had to cancel the cycle,' I tell him. 'The follicle hasn't grown. It isn't big enough.'

'Oh, sweetheart,' he sighs, stroking my hair. 'Shall we go and sit in the living room and you can tell me what you want to tell me. Do you want to talk? We can see if there is anything we can do to make you feel better.'

Bruce helps me to my feet and I love to feel his arm around me as we walk slowly into the room next door and sit down together.

'Would you like a glass of water? Or something stronger?' He smiles tentatively.

'Water's fine, thanks. You know, that felt as if it would never end. The pain...'

'It was a bit scary. How do you feel now?' he asks.

'I feel better – as if I've exorcised some ghost or something.' *I'm smiling. I haven't been able to smile for ages.*

★ ★ ★

Supper is comforting, cooked by Bruce and eaten on trays in front of the television. I feel ready to talk about the 'what now?' aspect of cancelling the cycle.

'I suppose I'll just have to get through next week and the week after that, to day one of the next cycle. It's strange, but I feel like I'm letting our child down; as if I am denying him a chance to come to us.'

Just then, a thought with a ray of hope attached to it enters my head: 'Now then. Wait a minute. My cycles alternate between 28 and 33 days, right?'

'If you say so,' replies Bruce.

'So, if that last cycle was a short one, and this is a long one, then surely you can't compare the follicles at this date and be sure that this follicle isn't going to grow at the last minute. This may just be a long, slow-growth cycle. What do you think?'

Bruce replies thoughtfully, 'I can see why you would think that. Do you think it's worth asking?'

'Well, we could pay for an extra couple of scans couldn't we? What would it be? Around a hundred pounds? Can we afford it?'

'Well, if it would reassure you one way or the other about cancelling or continuing, then I would say that it's worth it.'

Cycle two, day 16 – still no surge

At the clinic, I am put through to Brenda, who, thank goodness, is on duty again today. I tell her my thoughts, based upon my Slow-growing Follicle Theory.

'There's a chance I'm right isn't there? In theory? I respect your advice, but this follicle is on the unblocked side – I don't want to let it go if there is a chance of it growing to a good size.' I feel that I am hitting the right balance of respectful, but resolute.

'Well yes,' she replies slowly. 'It's possible. I'm still not convinced that this is a good enough cycle for you to continue. If it would put your mind at rest, of course you should book another scan.'

Seaside day trip

Thursday's scan, number four, was inconclusive because the follicle had only grown an almighty one and a half millimetres. The clinic has agreed to scan me again tomorrow, which is Sunday. Bruce will be able to come with me.

A while ago, we pencilled today into our diaries as a 'Day Out to the Seaside' to cheer ourselves up before the next insemination. We've decided to go anyway, taking our old camper van and Barney.

We've driven along the coast to Hayling Island and parked up by the sea. It's overcast, but we are having fun.

'It's going to be a laugh to all pile into the camper van for the weekend and lark about on the sands isn't it?' I can see us as a family very clearly in my mind's eye. 'Playing cricket on the beach, throwing balls into the sea for Barney. Yes honey, it'll all be worth it.'

Cycle two, day 19, scan five

As we arrive at the clinic, Bruce asks me, 'What are you expecting?' *I'm glad that he's not asking what I want.*

'Very good question, honey. I suppose that the worst thing would be an inconclusive result, like the one last Thursday. I want the decision to be made for me – no ifs or buts. Because the follicle is growing on the unblocked side, I just can't let this cycle go.'

It's a new sonographer; it must be Bridie's weekend off. This lady seems to be very kind. I haven't caught her name, but I can't be bothered to ask her to repeat it. I lie down and cover my knees with the blanket as she prepares the scan.

The screen is fuzzy blue-grey as usual, but there are no lines or black dents visible.

'Are we agreed that there are no follicles visible?' The sonographer now seems cold and unfeeling.

'What's happened?' I ask.

'I'm afraid that the follicle has collapsed. You haven't ovulated this month.' She is looking at me blankly. *That'll be why I didn't have a surge.*

'Oh. I see.' So that's it. The outcome I wanted. At least, that's what I thought. So why do I feel nothing, no relief, no resolution, nothing? I walk through to Bruce, who doesn't need to ask me the result. He puts his arm around my shoulder as we walk towards the door; he bids the receptionist 'goodbye' and 'thank you'.

'It was conclusive then?' he asks.

'Yes. Let's get home please. I'll be able to talk about it when we get home.'

12

Constructive communication

Cycle two, day 20

I have just arrived home from work, ready to discuss the next steps with Bruce this evening. As my ovulation was a non-event this month, I'm moving straight on to another cycle without taking a break. We have eight or ten days before I start my next period, so time is of the essence if I'm to discuss an improved treatment protocol with the doctors at the clinic. I'm not sure how much more of this I can take. And we're running out of money. We received a refund from the clinic as I didn't have the insemination, but we only have enough in the bank for one more try.

I hear Bruce's key in the front door and the sound wakes Barney, who pads off to meet him, pressing his nose against the doorjamb and inhaling loudly to confirm the familiar scent of his master.

'Is it Bruce? Is he home?' I scurry to the door, opening it before he turns his keys in the lock. Barney's tail is wagging so forcefully that his head is swinging backwards and forwards as well. I step back, letting him greet Bruce first. Barney has to reverse away from the door to allow it to open, but then pushes forward towards Bruce, who smiles broadly at both of us as he steps over the threshold.

'Is that my lovely family come to greet me? What a welcome home!' He leans down and kisses me softly on the lips, before pushing his large leather bag of artist's brushes and tools under the hallstand. We both follow Bruce through to the sitting room and Barney leaps up onto the sofa, placing a paw insistently on Bruce's thigh to get a tummy-rub.

'How's your day been, honey?' Bruce enquires, kissing my forehead as I lean down towards him.

'Not so good I'm afraid.'

Bruce looks concerned as he stops tickling Barney to hear how I am.

'I mean, work's good, it's a really supportive environment and not too taxing, but emotionally it's really hit me that my eggs are not what they were; that I am getting older. I suppose I accept the reality of the dramatic fall in fertility after the age of 38 that we were warned about. I may have been unrealistic in wanting this to happen quickly, and with no assistance from drugs.'

'Right,' says Bruce, in a tone that implies that he'd rather not be discussing this topic for the umpteenth consecutive night since my meltdown.

I press on. 'I want to skip a stage – move straight on to injections. What do you think?' I stop and take a sip of the water at my side to give him a chance to respond.

'What do you mean, "skip a stage"?' he asks.

'Well, the usual next stage is to use Clomid tablets – clomiphene citrate. It's a drug to induce ovulation. It tricks my body into producing more follicle-stimulating hormone and therefore more follicles. Injections are stronger, and they work in a different way. The drugs you inject are usually ovary-stimulating hormones or cycle-suppressing drugs used by doctors to give them more control over the treatment cycle. Even though they wouldn't need to harvest my eggs because we're not doing IVF, the drugs would still give me a better chance of developing a better quality and quantity of eggs.'

'Okay,' replies Bruce. 'But you said you didn't want to do injections.'

'But what if the tablets alone aren't enough to make me produce good enough eggs? We'll spend another thousand pounds or so and it may not work. We don't have enough money for more than one cycle. Also, you're totally fed up with all of this and just want to be a dad, so I think we should ask to move to stronger drugs and, yes...injections.' *I can't believe I'm suggesting this, but I just want to do as much as possible, as fast as possible, before I can't take any more.* 'It would be the best use of our funds and should reduce the time we have to spend trying to get pregnant. I'm thinking about getting back to normal as soon as we can – the longer I'm out of the live events scene, the harder it's going to be to get back in, especially if I'm lucky enough to have a baby. We've got to be realistic; I haven't been able to work to my full capacity since autumn last year; I've got to start pitching for decently paid management projects before this summer. I'm finding the lack of income as stressful as the treatment itself now.'

'I know what you mean; the pressure of being sole wage earner is not too hot either.' Bruce puts his arm around me. 'If you're sure about this, then let's go and discuss it with the clinic.'

Caro seems to be going through a thought process about our treatment while I'm out at work. I come home to see her visibly upset or saying 'I definitely can't do this, I can't stand this', or 'this isn't what I wanted', and we talk it round and round, eventually reaching some sort of resolution to continue or take a break, which all then changes again the next day. I honestly feel that I'm beginning not to care what we do, as long as we settle on something and see it through. I don't want to be wringing our hearts out every night, night after night reaching a decision to stop treatment for while, which changes again the day after. I'm beginning to find it exhausting.

'How are you feeling in other ways? Better?'

'Actually, these failures in my fertility have made me feel that I want to talk to someone...'

'And...?' asks Bruce.

I want us to see the counsellor together, but I don't think it's going to be well received. Here goes...

'I was thinking that it might help us to go to the clinic for counselling. We seem to be going through this in quite distinct and different ways. Counselling might help us to understand why.' *And now for my confession...* 'Actually, I've already booked an appointment. We can see Steve – do you remember him? He's the man who saw us for the mandatory sessions. He has a slot next Tuesday.'

'No, I don't think so,' Bruce snaps, removing his arm from around my shoulders. 'I've got you to talk to. It's your opinion I value; I don't feel a need to talk to a stranger about our private feelings.' He strides over to the bay window now, parting the wooden Venetian blinds and peering up and down the street seeking the source of a noise I haven't heard.

'That's not fair. That's too big a responsibility to put onto me as well as everything else.' I get up to go towards him, but find myself rooted in front of the sofa, unable to approach him. 'I don't understand my own feelings, even less know how to deal with the process you're going through,' I plead. 'Surely it would help us to understand what's going on, how to get back to how we were? I'm sure it will help. Please say you'll come.'

'No. I'm sorry. It's just not my thing. I feel that I've dealt with my diagnosis. It has been fairly conclusive after all.'

'You might be wrong. Are you *sure* you've dealt with it? I doubt it, to be honest. You seem to have taken this all so calmly.'

'Well, there isn't any point in being anything but calm is there; there's nothing we can do about it. The situation is the situation; talking about it isn't going to change anything.'

Dammit. I've caused a stand-off now. He's clammed up. I'll just have to go alone.

I'm just not going to get into this conversation right now. If she wants to go off and get counselling, that's up to her; but I don't. It's not going to help me at all. I don't think that we can talk any more deeply, or have any more insight into our particular situation, with a counsellor than we would have on our own here, at home. To be quite honest, I feel I have to be strong and objective for both of us and it's taking all my energy. I don't want to pick over the bones of my alleged insecurities with some stranger in the evenings. I don't feel insecure to the point of needing to talk about it. It's not my way of dealing with problems. I had no choice about the mandatory counselling, but I'm just not going to do this. I don't see the point.

Consultation and stimulated cycle

We saw Dr di Martino today, who has agreed to our request to move straight to 'the best chance', as she put it. We're on a high, feeling back in control of our treatment, and now in the consulting room with Clodagh, the nurse who first did Bruce's TESE procedure last year. It's nice to see a familiar face. She's going to teach us how to inject and take us through the information about the drugs we're using. She's giving a warning note about possible side effects.

'...nausea, mood swings, bloating. In the worse-case scenario, too high a dosage can lead to over-stimulation of the ovaries.'

'I couldn't take another cancelled cycle at the moment,' I say, but Clodagh reassures me.

'We don't usually have to cancel the cycle. It's more a question of resting up.'

'I'm fine about it, if you are,' says Bruce.

I look at Bruce. 'Will you do the injections? I can't face it. Do you mind? It'll make me feel more like we're in this together.'

'What if I hurt you?'

'You won't,' replies Clodagh. 'It's really easy. Honestly.'

She shows us two large, sealed, transparent bags: one contains syringes and needles, the other several packets of a drug called Merional. She tells us that it's an ovary-stimulating hormone to help my ovaries produce eggs. At her request, I take off my jeans and hop up onto the couch to expose my leg whilst she is unwrapping the hypodermic and syringe. The needle is very short and we're told that makes it easier for patients to self-administer. Diabetics use the same needles to inject themselves with insulin.

Bruce steps up to the mark, but hesitates before taking hold of the loaded syringe. Clodagh moves towards him as we all stare at my thigh.

'Now, you don't need to find a vein, the drugs only need to go in under the surface of the skin – subcutaneously.'

Bruce aims for my leg. 'Spot on,' says Clodagh, as Bruce injects me painlessly. I'm getting dressed whilst Bruce makes polite conversation with the nurse.

'Do you have any questions?' asks Clodagh, as I sit back down at the desk.

'Why did my follicles collapse and why didn't I get my surge even though I saw weak blue lines on my testing kit during the month?'

'Well, hormone levels fluctuate throughout the month. I'm afraid seeing evidence of them early on in the cycle is no guarantee that you'll ovulate.'

The more we learn about it, the fact that natural conception occurs at all is seeming more and more like a miracle.

'Well, let's hope it works for us this time,' says Bruce. He takes our drugs and needles from Clodagh. 'Ready for home, my lovely?'

Bruce picks up my jacket from the back of the chair and holds it out for me to put on. He turns my shoulders towards the door and we leave the clinic clutching our bags of equipment, paying for the next cycle on the way out.

Therapeutic counselling

I went for counselling last night. When I explained that Bruce hadn't wanted to come, Steve wasn't surprised – apparently it's very common. We talked about how different the responses of men and women are to infertility, especially when donor sperm are needed.

'It's quite common for men to focus on pushing through the treatment. It's an action – something that can be done to try to fix the problem. One of the most common negative effects of infertility in general is a sense of losing control. Focusing and driving through the treatment is one way of regaining that control.'

'But I've been trying to fix it for Bruce,' I reply. 'I don't know how connected it is, but one of my fears is that if I don't conceive, Bruce will eventually leave me.'

'But if you went,' Steve comments, 'he'd have to face starting a new relationship in full knowledge of his infertility. Coming to terms with being infertile from within a loving relationship is one thing, but telling a new partner about his circumstances would be quite a different challenge. It works both ways – both partners feel that they have a great deal to lose, even if they are not consciously aware of that.'

'But why am I having such a struggle dealing with the very treatment that may fix it for both of us? I have felt paralysed with fear, despair, anger. I just feel so depressed all the time.'

'Well, has it ever occurred to you that the child you have imagined, together with Bruce, the child you had a very strong sense of while you were chanting, was very real to you and that since Bruce's diagnosis, you've been dealing with a bereavement? You've been coping with the death of that child.'

So this is why I've been feeling so vulnerable, so raw. Steve tells me about other couples holding a private ceremony at home, or in a personally significant location, to say goodbye to the child they are not able to conceive. It helps them to find closure on unsuccessful treatment or miscarriage. He suggests that I find a way to say goodbye to our child.

To try to remove some of the strain I'm feeling, the counsellor encourages me to set a limit to the number of cycles I want to do and then stick to it. I have decided that this next one will be my last for now. Then I'll take a break before reviewing the situation in a few months' time.

Things not to say to an infertile couple

It was good to speak with someone who was sensitive and understanding. The most difficult part of this process of trying to conceive has been, and continues to be, dealing with insensitive comments and enquiries. Even when trying to support me by asking how I am, people tend to impose something of their own life story upon mine. I can spot the moment when they stop listening, searching their memory banks for something they see as comparable in their own life story. A triumphant expression crosses their face just before they jump in and offer some piece of advice, making *them* feel better instead of me.

I've made a note of some of the more unhelpful things people have said to us over the past months, and have analysed why they are, at worst, hurtful and, at best, well-intentioned but insensitive.

1. **'A friend of mine has had IVF treatment, so I do understand.'**

If you've said this, then I'm afraid that you probably don't understand. You have only understood as much as your friend has wanted you to know of her experience. The desire to have children is complex and so deeply ingrained in our biology that no one fully understands it until they meet a barrier to that desire. Moreover, there is an extra layer when speaking to a couple going through donor insemination, a layer of grief and anger that not only do they have to go through all of this clinical procedure, but that in the end the child they conceive will not be genetically connected to their loved one.

2. **'A friend of mine has been trying for years, and she has a baby now, so it's all been worth it.'**

Lucky friend. This doesn't help, and in fact merely serves to remind the unsuccessful couple of just how much of a failure they are. This also discourages the free choice to stop treatment, and makes us feel that we're under pressure to keep going and have 'just one more try'.

3. **'A friend of mine had IVF; as soon as she stopped she got pregnant.'**

This is an utterly pointless and thoughtless thing to say, especially if you have bothered to find out whether they are using donor gametes. If no sperm are present, no amount of making love will result in a pregnancy. Furthermore, don't assume that it's the woman who has the problem. Male factor issues are as common as female factors, and in some countries male factor problems are rising more rapidly. We are very tired of hearing about this 'friend' everyone seems to know who got pregnant naturally following the cessation of treatment, and we're beginning to wonder if everyone knows the same woman!

4. **'You just need to relax. It'll probably happen naturally.'**

You try relaxing when you are having to remember to take hormone tablets or have daily injections, visit a clinic every other day, keep count of the days of your cycle, pee on sticks for half the month, and watch out for dark-blue lines whilst you are still half asleep first thing in the morning! If I see my hormone surge, I have to drop everything the next day to have the insemination. Once you are 'going through' a cycle, the priority for that month has to be the treatment, but you cannot predict which days you will need the appointments, or indeed whether you will be able to have the treatment (unless you are having IVF, which has its own drawbacks), so you may well have cleared the month of appointments for nothing. This comment totally ignores the daily struggle of a cycle of fertility treatment. From Bruce's perspective, it is even worse. He deals with it by being very forthright in his response: 'Well, it's not going to happen naturally, because I'm infertile. So if we don't use donor sperm, perhaps you're suggesting that Caroline has an affair?'

5. 'Have you thought about adoption?'

You mean you can *adopt*? I'd never thought of that. Gee, thanks for your insight.

Adoption and fertility treatment require two different mindsets. Fertility treatment is a medical procedure leading to a pregnancy with a baby genetically connected to one or both of the parents. Adoption is the willingness to take on and raise someone else's child without having experienced a pregnancy. Examine your own reasons for having children, or adopting. Which would you prefer? It is important to allow a couple to say that they do not want to adopt without judging them or commenting on the children in the world who need homes – they already probably experience a measure of guilt about not feeling this way inclined. Adoption, by its nature, means that there are always other parents, council departments and agencies involved. Some couples just do not want to get involved in having children in this way, particularly since it is another lengthy and intrusive process.

7. 'You should join a mothers' group.'

I didn't understand this one at the time – and still don't. How would this help exactly? Bearing in mind the grief and sense of bereavement I've experienced, it feels cruel, like telling me to join a speed-dating club very shortly after being widowed.

8. 'I'll give you my kids for a day: you'll soon change your mind.'

We don't want *your* kids; we want our own. By saying this you are just rubbing salt into the wound. You are emphasizing your own proven fertility, while indicating that you are not grateful for this ability. Furthermore, this is usually said in front of the children, which can't do their self-esteem much good. This attempt at a light-hearted comment is never funny.

9. 'Have you tried...[assorted lists of vitamins/food supplements]?'

Tricky one this one, because it does come from a caring place, and from an appreciation of me wanting to achieve a pregnancy, and complementary therapies have shown good results in improving the success rates of pregnancy. But we can't afford them and I don't want to feel that I'm not doing something I should be. I have enough pressure already, both financial and social. Better perhaps to ask, 'I expect you've investigated all the foody things/complementary therapies available?' [Wait for response] 'Would you like me to let you know if I see anything interesting?' Or, 'I expect you've tried X Y Z? Any good?'

10. 'Gosh! I got pregnant without even wanting to!'

Mmm, not sure I need to explain why this is unhelpful.

11. 'Having children is not the "be all and end all" – it's bloody hard work you know.'

As if I didn't know this already. At our age, friends and relatives surround us with children. We shouldn't be judged for wanting what everyone else seems to have, and desiring what society seems to tell us is the ultimate achievement, and the source of true happiness. The people who say this normally already have kids of their own, so it just sounds patronizing. By opting for fertility treatment, we have been through a mandatory counselling programme and have considered the impact raising children will have on our lives, possibly more than a couple who can conceive naturally.

12. 'Isn't it funny how people who really want children can't have them, and others pop 'em out like shelling peas?'

This is not 'funny' at all – just a reminder of how unfair life can seem at times. You can change this to a helpful comment by emphasizing the apparent injustice and by appreciating our struggle by showing that you have noticed the irony of us being surrounded by people who are able to get pregnant with relative ease – including those who do so unexpectedly.

13. 'Maybe it's not meant to be.'

This has to be one of the most overused, supposedly compensatory phrases around. It is applied to anything that you want, have strived for, but are not achieving. To a person in pain, this is too big a leap to make. If we must, we will come to terms with our situation in time and perhaps even be happy being childless, but that is not for you to say. It is for us to decide.

14. 'The important thing is to keep focused on the aim of what you're doing.'

This is helpful in the early days, but as time and failed attempts pass, it is less helpful as it is inconceivable ('scuse the pun) that the couple are not focused on the aim of what they are doing – it is the only focus that is possible.

15. 'So has it worked yet?'

If we're not saying anything, it probably hasn't worked. A more general, gentle enquiry is likely to be more helpful.

16. 'I thought I might have received a phone call from you this year with good news.' [Said to us one year after our marriage by someone who knew we were having fertility treatment.]

Don't you think we'd be shouting it from the rooftops if a baby were on the way? Another friend said, 'We take it that no news is bad news,' which was much more helpful.

17. 'Never give up, Caroline.'

Unfortunately, whilst intended to be encouraging, this leaves me feeling as if I should struggle on trying and trying instead of being given the freedom to stop without fear of judgement. It increases the already huge pressure of the only successful outcome being one of achieving conception and pregnancy, rather than being free to come up with another solution – perhaps childlessness. Additionally, it implies that the person giving this advice has no idea about the financial, emotional and physical hardships imposed by fertility treatment. Why should the couple continue to put themselves through this?

I realize that before going through this experience, I too have been guilty of offering inappropriate advice, or of not listening properly. Now that I know how it feels to be on the receiving end, I will try to listen more carefully to others in the future. But for now, I just want to pull away from people who don't really understand.

I do have friends who have said good things as well. Here are the things that have helped.

1. **'I can't imagine how difficult this must be.'**

This is the best. It doesn't insult, or assume that you know how we feel, whilst showing that you care because you have given our situation some thought. It also allows us not to talk about it if we don't want to. A simple response can be, 'Thank you. It is awful/not so bad...'

2. **'How are you doing with the "baby stuff"/"baby project"? Or would you rather not talk about it?'**

If you are genuinely prepared for the couple not to want to discuss the current state of play, then this is also a very supportive question, as it lets them know that you are thinking of them and have not forgotten the ongoing situation, but want to take your cue from them. You are there if they need you, but won't pry.

3. **'How long have you been trying?'**

Again, this avoids insulting or undermining the perhaps already exhaustive efforts of the couple. I doubt whether someone who may have been trying for years and years has left many stones unturned. Let them talk. You may learn something!

4. **'Whatever the outcome, or whatever your decision, you have each other, and a loving relationship, and that's something special in itself. We know that you will be happy together, with or without children.'**

This, from our parents, removed one of the major longings of this experience – to give them grandchildren. We no longer felt as though we were letting them down, or that they were disappointed in any way, and it really helped.

5. **'Try to make each decision 100 per cent for yourself, and 100 per cent for each other.'**

This became the single most important and helpful method of reaching decisions. We were able to apply it to everything. It is easy in this process to feel that you should or ought to take particular action based on what you feel is expected of you, or is the 'right' thing to do, or what your partner really wants. *Don't do it if you are not happy to.* Check with yourself and with each other at every stage of the process. If it's the right decision, then you'll both be happy and resentment will not build up, nor will blame be apportioned unfairly.

6. **'Do what you can, while you can. That way, when you decide to stop, you will know that you did as much as you could, and you will have no regrets.'**

This has become so much a part of our decision-making process that I nearly forgot that once upon a time it was the advice of a friend. It is wonderful advice. It is not possible to know the future or predict outcomes, but if you are certain that you have done as much as you are able, or prepared, to do, then you are less likely to have regrets as time goes on – sadness of course (if things don't work out), but no regrets.

7. **'I have complete faith in you.'**

This was something said to me, by the counsellor at the clinic, at a point when I had completely lost faith in myself. The strength of a statement like this is immense. It made me dare to continue to believe in my own ability to make the right decisions and to see that I would, one day, feel strong again.

The bottom line is this: we would prefer people to ask us questions. Neither Bruce nor I mind talking about our experiences. We're trying to be open and honest; if we weren't, we'd have taken the decision to keep this a secret in the first place. Please engage brain before speaking and think about what you are going to say. Don't assume that you know how we feel.

If the basis for what you are about to say is 'I know what you're going through', then you're probably going to say the wrong thing. However, if the basis is 'You know your situation best' or 'No doubt you have thought about this more than I can begin to imagine', then your comment will probably be helpful and supportive.

Now, if only I can get pregnant...

13

Am I forcing Mother Nature?

The intensity and frequency of injections in a cycle mean living a six-week time period in a drug bubble. There is no choice but to let it overtake all other activities and normal daily existence. Paradoxically, although I have embarked on this next cycle out of choice, it feels as though choice – in terms of the ability to choose how to spend my days – has been taken away from me.

I still manage to go into work, thankful that I have flexible and part-time hours. Friends get in touch less frequently, as I can only talk about my treatment and the effect it has on me. At work, I 'm becoming increasingly withdrawn and distracted. I feel that I should be able to cope, but when I am writing entries in the diary I'm keeping so that I don't lose track of my treatment regime, I see how unhappy I am with my decision to put myself through this.

Bruce is working 12-hour days to keep us going financially. His tiredness combined with my increasing involvement with the treatment regime and solo ongoing counselling has meant that it's been really hard for us to connect. I am finding the counselling helpful; it helps me to gain insight into a male perspective in general, even if Bruce can't express what he's going through in particular. Bruce is not convinced it will help us, but I know that I need to understand my emotions more deeply in order to get through this. We both need to find ways to cope.

I'm taking these drugs in the hope that this will all be over as quickly as possible. Thank goodness that Bruce has agreed to give the injections to me – at least I feel as if we are experiencing this cycle together.

Cycle three, day 1

By my calculations, my period has arrived exactly 28 days after my previous one. Our child is evidently in as much of a rush to be here as I am to be pregnant. He or she is giving me the opportunity to get on with the next cycle very quickly after the disappointment of last month. I'm taking this as a good omen. It's going to work this time; I feel it in my heart. We *are* going to be parents.

Cycle three, day 3 – the first injection

Bruce having prepared the syringe at the dining table, with encouragement from me, we move into the sitting room so that I can lie on the sofa to expose my thigh to his hypodermic.

'Where shall I put it?' asks Bruce, nervously balancing the injection in his right hand, his thumb poised over the end of the plunger. I point to a site on my thigh, as we'd been shown at the clinic.

'Do it.' I encourage him by exaggerating my bravery and screwing my eyes tight closed. 'I'm ready.'

In it goes and out, almost without a sting. I'm relieved not to have to feign painlessness, as I don't want Bruce to come to dread the chore I've insisted on him executing.

'Okay?' he checks.

'Yes, fine. Honestly, I'm fine. It didn't hurt.' I smile at him whilst pulling my jeans up. I walk over to the fridge to see what I can prepare for supper, whilst Bruce packs up the needles in the special disposal pouches and then brings the bag of drugs to me to store in the cool box.

'When's the next one due?' he asks.

'The day after tomorrow,' I reply, closing the door with one hand, balancing a plate of cold ham with the other and walking to the kitchen. I'm trying not to trip over Barney, who is deliberating stop-starting and zigzagging in front of my shins as I walk, in the hope that he can trip me up and cause the meat to bounce off the plate and into his mouth.

Cycle three, day 4

I'm back at work today and it's a drug-free day. Bruce and I don't have to co-ordinate our movements or rush home to make 'the injecting hour'. Nurse Clodagh said that we must decide on morning, afternoon or evening timings for the injections and then try to stick to administering them at a regular hour.

Heather inspired me this morning during one of our support chats. We speak before I take Barney to the park and I've come to rely on her because she's practical and a good listener. She listens to what seem to me incoherent, inconsistent outpourings and somehow converts them into a pattern of behaviour or valid emotion. She invariably comes up with at least one action I can take to make me feel better. Baby steps; one step at a time to get me through each day. Today's topic is money and our rapidly dwindling coffers.

'How about renting out your spare room again? There may be a theatre tour in town. I can put a notice up at the stage door for anyone needing digs if you like.'

'Great idea. Thanks,' I reply.

The difficulty, of course, will be sharing the house with a stranger at a time when we need our privacy. All the same, it's a good plan, so we'll just have to close all the downstairs doors and hope we're not disturbed as the hypodermic is going in and I'm half-naked on the sofa.

Cycle three, day 5 – injection two

Bruce kept me awake most of last night with his snoring, so I'm exhausted. If I rent out the spare room, where will I go to escape his nocturnal rumblings? I suppose I'll have to get used to sleepless nights in the near future anyway, so it'll be good practice.

He's working late today, which causes a bit of an issue with the timing of the injection. I notice that no employment law protects couples *trying* for children. We've been dealing with this for nearly a year now, and it's getting harder. I've virtually closed down my business to accommodate the time I need; I can't work full-time and attend all the appointments. This treatment is hard enough in itself, even if I didn't have to work, but it's almost impossible if you need a double income, as I suspect is the case for most couples. From the financial perspective, I can only see things getting worse. Once I'm pregnant, Bruce is going to be sole wage earner for a while. We'll be starting our lives as parents from a weakened financial position, and that doesn't seem very sensible to me.

The second injection into my thigh was a little sore tonight.

Cycle three, day 7 – injection three

I can't believe how debilitating this is turning out to be. The effect of the hormone treatment is very subtle: external circumstances don't trigger my mood swings; it all happens spontaneously from within. I slip in and out of good and bad moods without noticing the transition. It has the effect of making me feel that I must be going slightly crazy. The bad mood feels real, but when I try to find a reason why I'm irritated by people or events, I can't. I exist behind a layer of padding – suffocating underneath a duvet insulating my face, brain and body. I can't discard it no matter how hard I try.

Today, as I passed the walk-in stationery cupboard at work, I stopped to say hello to a colleague from a different department. She was busy, but noticed that I looked a bit down in the dumps, so asked how I was feeling. To my surprise, she wasn't just being polite, but really wanted to know. I told her the truth.

'The mood swings and nausea are killing me. It's really hard to concentrate and focus on the detail of what I'm doing. I didn't expect to react to the drugs this quickly; I had hoped not to experience any side effects at all.'

'Ah yes, I remember that feeling from when I was pregnant with my boys.' She has two sons, now aged three and five. She tells me that the change in your body and mind is subtle, the pregnancy hormones are subtle; she uses the word 'insidious'. So it's not just pregnancy that can make you feel rough, but *pregnancy hormones* too. I find it ironic that I now have something in common with pregnant women – so near and yet so far.

I've often heard friends with children comment on how their self-confidence is affected by pregnancy and motherhood. I'm finding that my self-esteem is being eroded with each and every failure, and that this is pervading other areas of my life. Somehow, because I'm failing to get pregnant, I'm beginning to think that any prior successes I've had in my career or in my relationships are insignificant compared to the ability to fulfil my 'fundamental function' as a woman. But how can success possibly be connected to pregnancy? It doesn't make sense. The ability to become pregnant isn't connected to whether you are deserving of being a parent, or to whether the baby is planned, unplanned, wanted or not. It's all pretty random, or so it seems to me.

★ ★ ★

This evening brought a telephone call and visit from a touring theatre sound engineer who would like to stay until March. Perfect timing. He found us via Heather's theatre contacts. He seems really nice and very considerate, but sharing the house with lodgers is not going to be easy when Bruce and I are going through something so private. I hope I can keep my moods in check.

We tried a different jab site for the third injection tonight – into my belly. Bruce prepared the syringe on his own, in the conservatory, because I felt tense at the thought of watching him do it. Going into my belly was better than into my thigh.

Cycle three, day 8 – no injection

I wonder if this extra stimulation of my ovaries will lead to twins? They run in my family. Mum has always teased me that they have now skipped a couple of generations. I'd love to have twins. I know it would be really hard work, but at least having two babies at once would mean that I don't have to go through this again and we won't run out of time to have more children. Back in the 1960s, my father, ever the cautious doctor, discouraged my mum from having any more because of the potential health risks of being an older mother. She was only 35 when I was born – but still termed an 'elderly primigravida' on her notes. How off-putting.

I broke down in tears again tonight. I cry so much these days that I have learned to sob quietly so as not to wake Bruce. If he wakes and asks me what's wrong, I struggle to find a definite reason. I just cry.

Obviously I have to continue with the cycle I'm on at the moment, and with these damned drugs, which are making me feel so rotten, so I'm going to sit down in front of Gohonzon, the focus for my Buddhist chanting, and try to connect with the spirits of our babies – conjure up a vision of them as best I can. I'll tell them that this is their last chance to come to us. Bruce says that we are doing all that we can, and now it's up to them.

Cycle three, day 9 – injection four, first scan

There are a few tiny follicles showing up on the right-hand side, which is the one that might be blocked. It's so frustrating. When I was tested originally, my FSH levels were better than expected for my age, but now it seems that my follicles and uterine lining are in a worse than expected state. This makes me realize that hormone levels are not necessarily connected to the activity in my ovaries.

I have to increase the frequency of the injections to boost my cycle even more. Bruce must give me an injection every night until Saturday, then I'm booked in for a scan on Sunday, and probably another one on Tuesday. Monitoring for my surge with the ovulation testing kit begins on Monday – day 13 of this cycle. After that, I have to test every morning for five days, so the next fortnight to three weeks is completely screwed. We were hoping to book a holiday, but we can't; we've been invited to France on a day trip, which would be lovely and remind us of more carefree times, but we can't do that either. Taking into consideration the side effects I'm experiencing, I can't even risk inviting friends round for dinner, or to meet for a drink, because I can't predict how I'll be feeling from one day to the next.

I had an 'attack of the side effects' this afternoon in fact – I'm grumpy without reason, nauseous and headachy. I feel the sickness coming on in a wave and have to lie on the sofa until it passes. I'm really fed up – fed up that we are infertile, really annoyed and frustrated. This process is not for me, but how can I stop when we haven't been able to give it a good shot yet? The injections hurt now. The nurse said cheerily, 'Oh, you'll get used to them.' I won't. Is it all worth it?

I'd always assumed that I could have children whenever I was ready, seduced into thinking that this is my right as a woman. Loads of other women are doing it, and there's no history of sub-fertility in my family, so I must be able to get pregnant. I think the impact on your life of finding that you are apparently unable to achieve a lifelong desire is generally underestimated. It has become my focus, and I'm sacrificing so much to pursue it. I wish the clinic had warned us how challenging this was going to be. Why isn't there more information available about the financial and projected timeline aspects of the treatment? If there were, maybe I'd have been able to make better-informed choices. It would be useful to include a 'financial prospects' element in the mandatory implications counselling alongside the legal and emotional parts. We needed to think about the effect of losing one of our incomes having just paid for a wedding and bought a family home. I know that children are expensive, but at least couples blessed with the ability to conceive naturally have nine months to make plans, and to budget once pregnant.

Unable to receive treatment on the NHS, and unwilling to go abroad, we are left with no choice but to spend enormous amounts even to get to 'first base'. Thinking back, the clinics have been totally upfront about how much each cycle costs, but what they can't tell us is how many cycles I may need, or how long we may be struggling. The side effects I've been experiencing mean that I can't possibly contemplate pitching for event management contracts, which continues to impact on my earning capacity. Every woman I've spoken to confirms that life goes on hold, both during and after the treatment, whether or not you end up pregnant. That's better. Rant over – for the moment.

Cycle three, day 10 – injection five

There's hope for me yet. I have just heard on the grapevine that not one but *two* women I know – one from my theatre days and one of my neighbours – are pregnant for the second time, naturally, at 43. They both had their first babies at 41, older than I am now.

Cycle three, day 11 – injection six

I wonder if we can harvest extra eggs from this cycle and use them to move straight on to IVF next month? I wouldn't have to endure as many drugs or another month feeling as grotty as this. I'll check with the clinic tomorrow when I go for my scan.

Cycle three, day 12 – second scan

There's good news and bad news. The good is that there is now a follicle on the left. It's small, because of my long cycles, and it's growing slowly, but it *is* growing. I'm with Nurse Jameela, who is analysing the notes from my latest scan.

'I understand from Bridie, the sonographer, that you're finding the treatment a bit of a struggle and want to take a break after this one.' *Bridie must've been fighting my corner – that's nice.* 'Well, I've spoken to the professor, as your consultant is on holiday, and he has agreed to let the cycle continue.'

'Why? Was there a doubt?' I ask.

'The follicle is small; we would usually recommend cancelling and waiting for more significant growth – between 15 and 17 millimetres. We're going to increase the dosage and frequency of your injections to encourage development, but this is only because you've elected not to cancel. Please bear in mind that you're going to continue to feel grotty for the rest of the month. You can still cancel if you prefer…'

'Well, with a bit of luck and more drugs, I should be returning with nice juicy follicles in a few days. Then I can go ahead as planned.' I thank Jameela and book another scan. *I had no idea I might have to abandon the second cycle in succession. That would have been a disaster.*

I hope I am doing what's right for my life. During my time spent chanting, I have explored what it would be like not to have kids, almost succeeding in talking myself out of all of this torture. As a result, the thought that it might work is also scary, especially as I feel now that I'm taking risks I was formerly not happy to take. I often think of the promise I made to Barbara about not doing anything I didn't want to do, but I've changed my mind. I'm not betraying my promise, just doing what I must do to get pregnant.

★ ★ ★

We had a little time to kill this afternoon before we had to be home to do the next injection. We went looking at cars, as a diversion as much as anything. We felt slightly stymied because we don't know whether we are looking for a family car or something more economical and compact. Bruce tried to cheer me up by saying we should get a silly sports car as compensation if this cycle doesn't work. My car is so old, but I have to rely on our local garage to keep it limping on for a while longer.

Cycle three, day 13 – Clearplan testing day 1, injection seven

I didn't sleep well last night; it took until the early hours to drop off – at about two o'clock I think. There's a great deal of tension in my body. I had a dream that I'd peed on the Clearplan stick without noting the result and that I'd gone out for the evening without taking my stick with me. I wish this were over.

Cycle three, day 14 – Clearplan testing day 2, scan three

The scan didn't show much change – nothing conclusive to say whether or not the follicles have perked themselves up a bit.

Bruce and I got it together to make love this morning, sort of. It was quite uninspiring for both of us, unfortunately, but at least it went a little way towards making us feel human again.

Cycle three, day 15 – Clearplan testing day 3, no injection

I feel this morning like a big egg, or an old Friesian cow pumped full of hormones. This is so undignified. I had my second counselling session today. The sessions are definitely helping to restore a little of my confidence. I said I felt at times as if I was losing my mind. I've never felt this intense before. The counsellor reassured me that my feelings are as valid as anyone else's: 'They are your feelings and therefore they are valid.' I had a bit of a breakthrough about what using donor sperm means to me. It is just the means by which our child will come to us; the donor sperm is just a means of transport. Our baby *has* always been and *will* always be our child. I don't mean that I'm not grateful to the donor; I am. Without his altruism we wouldn't have even had this chance.

Cycle three, day 16 – Clearplan testing day 4, scan four

I've just had the final scan of this cycle. There are four large follicles – two on each side. I've had my surge, so we've come to the clinic to collect the injection to trigger ovulation. Bruce is with me, as it's Saturday and he's not working, and we're now waiting for Jameela to give us the 'all clear' to schedule the insemination. It feels like the opening night of a new show! But then I remember the implications of having more than one dominant follicle. Clodagh warned us about ovarian hyper-stimulation syndrome, or OHSS. I'm assuming I'm all right so far, because the nausea hasn't been serious – debilitating certainly, but not frightening; I haven't actually been vomiting. But I know that with four follicles present I run the risk of a multiple pregnancy.

'If all four follicles are released by the trigger injection,' I ask, 'does that mean that all four may be fertilized by the donor sperm?'

'Yes, that's right.'

'So, if all four are fertilized…'

'Yes. There is a possibility of quads,' she says. 'That's why we were considering cancelling the cycle. But you've been told about the possibility of reduction if that occurs?'

Clodagh mentioned reduction and gave us some information leaflets after she taught us how to inject. We were warned that more fertilized eggs can result in a multiple pregnancy. In my case, if all four of my follicles develop into embryos, the clinic will advise a reduction to twins in order to give two babies the best chance of going to full term and being healthy. The process of reduction involves injecting potassium into the heart of the most easily reached foetus (or foetuses) in the womb, which is then absorbed back into the body.

Just as we are about to leave, it occurs to me to ask, somewhat as an afterthought, if they could double-check that our donor code was still that of the French doctor. Jameela checks the code in our file, on the notes for this month, and then turns back to the charts for our previous insemination.

'Oh. You've been re-coded. They must have run out of stock from your last donor.'

'What?' I ask. 'How can this happen without our knowledge?'

'Don't worry,' Jameela reassures us. 'Let me call the cryolab and see why they've done it.'

She leaves the room as I whisper to Bruce, 'What a good thing I checked.' He nods in agreement and takes hold of my hand under the desk. Jameela returns a few minutes later, with good news.

'You'd been re-coded because the lab is running low on stock from your previous donor. But there is some left, so I've reserved it for you.' She adds a note of caution: 'You probably won't be able to return for a full sibling for your child. That's the reason we try to ensure that there is as much as possible of the same stock available.'

Returning for a sibling in the future. I can't even think past this experience, let alone consider coming back in a few years for more.

★ ★ ★

Bruce gave me the trigger injection at exactly eight o'clock in the evening, as instructed. The timing has to be precise for the insemination to have the best chance of success.

'Release the follicles!' he cried triumphantly, and hummed a little of the 'Dambusters' theme tune. I had to stifle my laughter for fear of putting him off his stride with the needle. We've come this far, and I'm delighted that there are no more injections – whatever happens. Now I just have to chant for success.

Cycle three, day 17

At about five o'clock this morning I started to have horrendous stomach cramp, which grew steadily worse until dawn, when it gradually died away. It must have been the follicles being released. I'm feeling a bit tender around the abdomen just now, but very excited. I'm really looking forward to this working well and to the excitement and challenge of being pregnant, but this has definitely taken its toll on my psyche. I had two horrible nightmares last night: in one a stranger was repeatedly sexually assaulting me, and in the other I was carrying triplets, two boys and a girl, and the girl triplet was disintegrating inside me – I could actually feel it – and had to be removed by surgeons to save the two boys. It was awful.

If I'm lucky enough to conceive twins, I'll take great care of them. They just have to find the small space inside me where they can snuggle down for nine months. I'll do the rest. Actually that's not true: they're going to have to do their bit too – we need some teamwork here.

Insemination day

The big day has arrived at last. Bruce is with me, but we've decided not to repeat our last experience by trying to imbue the procedure with fake intimacy or romance. Bruce brings a book and takes a seat downstairs in the waiting room. I follow the nurse upstairs. Making a minimum of fuss feels more acceptable.

It's the same routine: 'Feet in the stirrups please. Try to relax', sperm in fluorescent pink fluid, catheter in, cramping, catheter out and finish. Now follow 14 days of torture before we know whether or not it's worked.

After the insemination, I'm warned again about multiple births and advised on foetal reduction. As we walk back to the underground, heading for home, Bruce asks, 'What do you want to do if it fails again, honey?' I understand why he's asking this apparently defeatist question – no doubt he wants to prepare for the emotional meltdown that may follow. It must be so hard for him to guess what I'm thinking; I'm confused in my own mind, so it must be doubly difficult for him on the outside of my thoughts. I've tried to be nonchalant about the outcome of this cycle; tried to be ambivalent about the result. I don't want to build our hopes. For the sake of our relationship, I've said we'll take a break if this one doesn't work.

However, my response to his question is an emotional u-turn: 'I want to carry on with treatment until we get a baby or bab*ies*.' *Where did that come from? I sound emphatic, but I certainly don't feel it.*

'Why the change of mind? You've been so resistant to the idea during the ordeal of this last cycle.'

I try to come up with a reasoned explanation for how I'm obviously truly feeling deep inside: 'I think that we've come so far and now that I've done what I promised never to do, by having injections, we may as well push on until we have succeeded in having our child. "Failure is not an option," as they say. I'm really determined to be a mum.'

Caro is far more vehement than I about whether or not to continue. To an extent, I'm just happy to go with what she wants to do, but with either scenario there's a big implication for me. If we carry on, I have to be kind to her, deal with the mood swings and try my best to keep earning money. If it works this time, then I know that there are bound to be nights when I get back from work and she'll be clambering the walls, having dealt with small babies or children all day whilst I've been out at work. Perhaps this is down to a difference in the way men and women deal with problems: I don't seem to hang on to things, or need to analyse them in the way that Caroline does. Ultimately, I just want her to be happy with whatever she chooses to do.

Cycle three, day 1 of the two-week wait

I called a friend of mine who has IVF triplets. He laughed when I asked him how he and his wife cope with their two girls and a boy, now 13 years old.

'Well it's a challenge for sure. When we had IVF there was no limit on how many embryos were put back in the uterus. It was early days for assisted conception.'

'Did they talk to you about reduction?'

'Yes, of course. But they gave us the alternative of my wife taking bed rest in hospital for the final three months of her pregnancy.'

'So you never contemplated losing one of them?'

'Well, I know that it's much safer to reduce, and the advice is good, but we decided to take the risk. After all that effort to get pregnant, all the heartache and worry of getting them through the first trimester, we just couldn't do it.'

'Logically, it's the only safe advice the doctors can give I suppose – better to have fewer, healthy live births than not reach the end of a pregnancy you've dreamed of. I don't think I could agree to reduce, but there must be other couples who don't have a choice for financial or medical reasons. I'd better chant for twins I think.'

My friend wishes me the best of luck and offers a listening ear whenever I need one. I feel more certain of what to do should all four follicles fertilize: bed rest and prayer; hope and courage.

Cycle three, day 2 of the two-week wait

I could be two-and-a-bit weeks pregnant by now. I'm in high spirits. I'm a little closer to getting back to well-paid work and renewed, if temporary, independence (once I've got over the morning sickness of course).

Cycle three, day 3 of torture fortnight

I have pains in my stomach today. I've been given progesterone tablets to take for the next fortnight, to encourage implantation. This is making me feel as sick as the first drug. Everyone keeps telling me that all this nausea is 'a good sign' and that they are really excited. I'm not excited; I just feel ill. It's really tough. There's no point in being excited until after I'm 12 weeks pregnant, which will be mid-May. I'm trying to rest. I realize that you have to plan to take five or six weeks out of your life each time you go for a cycle.

Cycle three, day 4 of torture fortnight

I worked a short day today, as I only managed four hours before I had to go home feeling achy and nauseous. I have a really gripey stomach. Apparently it's the Progynova I'm absorbing in pessary form. It's a progesterone-type drug to encourage implantation. I can't work normally at all.

Cycle three, day 9 of torture fortnight

It's been a very difficult weekend. I've ricocheted between 'It's okay if I'm not pregnant' to the exact opposite view, and I feel this morning as if I'm going to get the mother of all periods, with cramping and breast tenderness. Maybe that's why I'm talking myself out of wanting this to work – because I don't think it has. I'm keeping my fears to myself, just in case I've been lucky. I've tried sharing my doubts with friends, but everyone tells me not to be negative. Bruce understands, but there's a limit to how much I feel it's fair to talk to him about this endlessly stressful process.

If I *am* pregnant, I need acknowledgement and understanding from my friends and family of the effort it's taken. If I'm *not* pregnant, I need acknowledgement and understanding from them of how hard I tried.

Cycle three, day 11 of torture fortnight

I saw spots of blood today. If it's a good sign, it certainly doesn't feel like one. I feel as though I'm not pregnant. I won't pre-judge it until Saturday, but if I'm not pregnant, I don't understand why not. I would make a good mother, so what's the point of my not having children?

I have gained something from this experience: I am stronger. I have proved that I can be patient and that I'm tenacious and determined. If I'm not pregnant, I want the perfect job, a great job that will enable me to make a difference in the world.

If we carry on, we have to find the funds – and I have to find the willpower. I do now understand why people keep going: it's a dogged determination. This process has nothing to do with making love or being together with your lover.

Cycle three, day 12 of 14

Although the bleeding had stopped by the time I went to bed last night, it has started again this morning. Barbara, with whom I now walk in the park on a regular basis, said the bleeding could be a sign of implantation, which really cheered me up. I spoke to a nurse at the clinic, who told me that the symptoms of implantation and menstruation are very similar: cramping and spotting. They are also individual to each woman, depending on her individual period pattern, and that at day 12, the pregnancy hormone, human chorionic gonadotrophin (hCG), wouldn't show up. This is so frustrating.

I'm trying to feel grateful for this opportunity to work on my impatient nature.

Cycle three, day 13 – the day before the pregnancy test

It's so hard to keep going. It's 24 hours too early to do the pregnancy test, but I am still bleeding. It's not a flow, it just keeps stopping and starting, but it's getting heavier.

All I want is for Bruce and me to be parents – to care for our baby, a baby I've been pregnant with and given birth to. Nothing else will do. Everything else pales into insignificance – I want this so badly. Cathy and Oyin came round to chant with me this evening. They encouraged me to remain optimistic, but when I pointed out to them my typical pre-period acne on my face and told them about the bleeding, even they struggled to stay upbeat.

Pregnancy test day

I had to do a test at 5.35 this morning because I needed a pee and I test the first one of the day. I didn't wake Bruce; it seemed unfair, as he had to be up for work at six o'clock. I was half asleep, but even so I could see that it was definitely negative. But I'm not bleeding properly yet. I also have a head cold now, so I'm feeling very sorry for myself.

Cycle three – day after two-week wait

I was still holding on to the hope that the negative pregnancy test could have been wrong, but there's no denying that the blood I'm seeing is my period starting properly. I can't understand why my period is more than a day late if I'm not pregnant. I'm calling the clinic to get more information.

'Hello. Could you put me through to the nurses' station please?' The line goes dead for a moment. Jameela answers and I explain my situation. Jameela tells me that the progesterone I have taken to spruce up my womb lining will have delayed my period. I plunge into despair. I can't think what to do, until I remember Steve's advice about finding a way to say goodbye to the child we can't have. Perhaps I still haven't let go.

I decide that one way of communicating my feelings could be through writing a letter to my fantasy child.

My boy,

You're there. I can really feel you. Sometimes I can see you. When I think about you, I can't make the decision I may have to make – not to give you, or any other babies, life – our 'default position', as Bruce calls it.

'Come on, Mum, hurry up. It'll be FUN.' That's what you said to me.

I've tried to hurry up, but I can't go on much longer. My energy to keep going is diminishing; I'm losing my will and my fight. The parts of me that would be fun for you are receding as I am gradually overwhelmed by sadness at not being able to make you appear as my own flesh and blood.

I wish I could forget you. Make a decision, and move on. But I can't seem to do that. You're there in my head and in my heart. If I turn away from you to live my own selfish life, surely I'll regret it. It feels like murder, or at least the denial of life; you never had a chance to be born.

Lately, I've seen two other children – a boy and a girl. They are gentle souls. My twins. They've been in the background, waiting for their chance. Perhaps they can't be mine until I've really kissed you goodbye.

Who are you really? You urge me on, but you also hold me back. Are you all literally our children? Or are you new ideas, waiting for me to jump back into life, grasp my potential and run into the future, the way maybe Nature intended, without children? After all, before these treatments were available we'd have had to be satisfied with being a childless couple, or maybe adopting.

But I want a child of my own; to be pregnant and give birth, even if I can never give life to Bruce's child. You are all meant to be ours; I feel it. I feel you out there. Please help me. Either be here, or leave me alone. Come to me, or fade away and allow me to stop this treatment.

14

'I don't mind what we do, as long as we decide something'

I no longer know what to do in order to get the best outcome for us. I want to stop, but that means no children – ever. Where would that leave Bruce and me? We've opened up this baby-shaped hole in our lives. We have explored what it should look like, feel like, to be parents. How do we ever close that hole again and carry on as before?

Should I give it another try? The trouble is I don't know if I can withstand the process yet again. But what if doing nothing is the wrong decision? Will I regret that forever? Even if I don't, will Bruce blame me at some point in the future when it's definitely too late to change our minds? A knot in my stomach has now developed, which, I admit, makes a change from the cramping. I keep making decisions, then panic and change my mind once more.

Even my usual processing method and path to enlightened action is proving unfruitful. I've been feeling that chanting isn't doing much good in my life at the moment. My faith no longer seems to be providing the support I need. But if I'm honest, I know that's not true. It's really helped me to know my own mind and decide what extra support I need. I ring Sanda to get her 'take' on my doubts.

'I think you need to decide what true happiness means to you,' she says, 'instead of what you think it *ought* to mean according to social expectations and your upbringing. Have the courage to examine your desires more deeply.'

As a result of this advice, I decide to go upstairs and chant for one hour. As I search for answers, I think about better times. When I worked in the entertainment industry, my life felt exciting and fulfilling.

From the age of 12, I wanted a career in the theatre. Not as an actor, but as one of the 'backroom boys', as they were termed – stage management, costume, or stage crew. My mother had taken me to see big West End shows from an early age. I saw my first production aged six in 1970: *Mame*, starring Frankie Vaughan and Ginger Rogers. I asked her if we could sit, not facing the stage head on, but off to one side of the auditorium where I could perhaps see into the wings, to catch a glimpse of how the magic was being created.

My first professional theatre job came through two contacts, now lifelong friends, Julie and Andrew, who already worked at our local repertory theatre. Julie advised me to keep badgering the stage manager for work until she was so sick of speaking to me that she'd give in and employ me. I kept this up for nearly a year until my persistence paid off. I was employed as a follow spot operator for the pantomime. On the first day of technical rehearsals, I walked up to the stage door. I was 17 years old.

'I'm here to see the stage manager for *The Wizard of Oz*. I'm Caroline Nicholson.'

Andy arrived from backstage to collect me and I passed through the double swing doors, off limits to the general public. There was a strange and lovely smell in the brown-and-faun-painted corridors and a sense of energy that I came to crave and which I now miss dreadfully. I felt that I had come home. This was where I was meant to be. It was magical, challenging and special – the camaraderie, the sense of fun coupled with a mission of creating something for the delight of an audience.

So what has happened to my world? Where did it go? Whatever happened to that confident, ballsy girl who wouldn't give up until she succeeded? She got the stuffing knocked out of her, that's what happened. Someone recently congratulated me on remaining motivated and optimistic throughout the fertility treatment, but it's all an illusion – the true nature of my new life is a three-act tragedy, playing itself out quietly in the wings, not on show to the public. If anyone asks, I usually reply that I'm fine, but then can't back up my statement.

I still get invitations from theatre mates to watch rehearsals and previews. I saw a wonderful opera dress rehearsal the other morning. In my randomly selected single seat, I was sitting next to someone I know who is working on the show currently playing in the venue where I used to work – the world-famous Royal Albert Hall. Two seats across in the other direction

I spied my design tutor from drama college, but decided I was feeling too shy to say hello. At the interval I scuttled away to find a quiet corner of the coffee bar, but I bumped into my first boss from repertory theatre. I felt comfortable talking to him; he and his wife were some of the best and most supportive bosses I have ever worked for. He filled me in on news of his family and of my former colleagues, but then I stumbled as he asked me what I was doing these days. I couldn't think of a benign excuse quickly enough and ended up revealing the real reason why I was 'taking a break' from my chosen profession, to the embarrassment of both of us.

I *liked* me when I worked in the entertainment industry. What did I like about myself? Well, I laughed a lot, and I made other people laugh. I was highly professional and I would get a buzz from listening to the requirements of the project, assessing the obstacles to success, and then sorting it, making sure everyone was happy – bringing intractable problems under control, making the impossible a reality, on time and on budget.

But I've changed. Now I hide in the shadows, in pain and regret. I don't sleep well and I frequently have dreams in which I've failed at some job or other. By my standards, I'm not successful any more, and seem to be playing my life in a minor key. I'm exhausted. If it weren't for my saviour Barney the dog getting me out into the park each morning for his walk, I doubt that I'd get out of bed or bother to get dressed at all.

Every time I reach a new low, I believe I can't go any lower, that I've turned the corner. But it's not true. I'm heading right now for the deepest low ever. I have to believe that it is darkest just before the dawn; that I am close to breaking through. I'm not doing what I want to do, not doing what I'm trained to do, not earning any money – and all because I wanted a baby.

I bring my chanting to a close by sounding the large bell beside me. Having faced my demons and admitted to myself how disappointed I am, I feel better. I'm ready to explore the relatively uncharted territory in my counselling session this evening.

Post-insemination counselling session

Steve is sitting opposite me in the primrose-yellow counselling room. I'm trying not to fiddle with the fronds of the palm tree that stands in a large pot to my left.

'My feelings are so confused. I don't know who I am or what I want any more. But I'm here, so I need to know how best to deal with the situation. I don't know what I want to do.'

Steve tries to comfort me by saying, 'You're a 40-year-old woman who wants a child. It's a very powerful biological urge. I don't think you need to analyse your desire any more than that.'

I relax for the first time in days. 'I'm fighting Nature then. Is that what you're saying?'

'Absolutely,' replies the interpreter of my emotions. 'Please don't punish yourself for having perfectly normal feelings. Our bodies want us to procreate, and if you are not seeing results for your enormous efforts, that's bound to be stressful.'

'But what about the erosion of my confidence? Why can't I pull myself together? Why do I feel so panicky? I'm scared that if I take time to explore my feelings now, take time to feel relaxed and ready to try again, I may leave it too late. I know that I'm running out of time, but I don't feel ready to do another cycle – nowhere near.'

Steve encourages me with options: 'You do have a little more time if you consider IVF or donor egg and sperm.'

'I don't even want to talk about that option thank you.'

'Why not?'

'Because the drugs made me so sick, and I assume that the amount I would need for IVF would only make things worse. And the cost...'

Steve looks at me a little sternly over the top of his half-rim spectacles. 'Okay, but I still think it would be a good idea to remember that the success rates are so much higher than for IUI. I know that money is an issue for you, as it is for many patients, but financially it's the best option, as there's more chance of success, and if you want to explore everything, you shouldn't miss out an entire stage.'

This gives me food for thought and I agree to talk about IVF in our next session.

Steve adds, 'You could always make an appointment with Mrs Storry and discuss the possible outcome of IVF in your particular case. You don't need to feel pushed into anything.'

'Okay, I'll think about it. Thanks.'

To my relief, the topic is closed until further notice. As we wind up the session for the evening, he compliments my courage and reassures me that we are making progress. I'm grateful for someone to talk to like this. Bruce seems to be getting increasingly weary of discussing my angst and indecision.

Reviewing my feelings

Bruce has to work today, so I've taken the opportunity for a girly chat with Marianne. What would I do without good friends – she and Heather have always been there for me, and now that commitment has become my lifeline.

'Is the kettle on?'

'You must have heard it boiling!' she says, welcoming me into her home with a big bear hug. We begin to talk as she makes the coffee in the mugs I bought for her some years ago as a birthday gift. 'So, how have you been matey?'

'You and I have known each other so many years…,' I begin.

'From primary school to now, an unbelievable 33 of them,' she interrupts playfully. 'But I don't look a day older and neither do you.'

'Am I doing the right thing, trying to have this baby for Bruce and me?'

Marianne sits down at her kitchen table. I follow her with my drink.

'With Bruce, you have found something that most people never find. He's your best friend, your lover, your confidant; you're so good together.'

'I know, but we're not as close as we used to be; we don't seem to be able to connect in the same way.'

Marianne continues: 'Most couples feel that having a child will bring them closer together, but this process seems to be driving you further apart. Do you think you could be jeopardizing your happiness by doing another cycle? It seems to me that you're missing out by putting yourself through this. Sorry if that seems a little harsh.' She takes a sip of coffee, placing it carefully down on one of the coasters we made for her last Christmas.

Certainly, Bruce and I don't hold hands walking along the street as we used to; holidays are becoming a distant memory because of the expense; we're not even going out to the movies any more, because by the time the weekend comes around, he's too exhausted to want to go anywhere.

'I suppose I feel that it's still early days for our relationship. I want to go travelling with him and Barney. I certainly want to get our sex life back to normal…'

I see my friend's surprise and concern as she stops drinking her coffee. I nod confidentially. 'We're both having difficulties in that department.' I don't think she realized, although I'm sure that she can't be surprised. 'Maybe, subconsciously, I'm resisting, even *preventing*, this happening.'

'Maybe you don't really want a baby at all – it's just something you feel you *should* do; that it's always been expected of you.'

I can't accept what Marianne has just said. 'I think it's good to be examining my motives, *but* I don't think that's true. For a start, even when I worked in the theatre I was in what I thought was a stable relationship. I was engaged shortly after I left drama college. It didn't work out because he didn't share my desire to have children. Oh, by the way,' I remember, 'did I tell you, he and his wife now have *two* sons? We met up at a wedding recently.'

'You hadn't told me. That must sting.'

'No, not really. He wasn't the right man for me. If we hadn't split up, I may never have met Bruce, so I count my blessings really.'

'Absolutely,' she agrees.

I continue: 'Bruce and I didn't intentionally make the decision to leave having children late; we thought we were being responsible.'

'No, well it's the same for lots of couples isn't it? What with busy careers, getting on the property ladder and meeting the right partner.'

Marianne changes the subject: 'How's the counselling going? Is it helping?'

'Yes, it's definitely helping me. But Bruce won't come with me, so there you go.' I shrug my shoulders.

Talking to Marianne has helped a little, but by the time I leave her house I still don't how to connect with Bruce, or whether having counselling alone is doing us more harm than good. All I know is that it's helping me. Bruce is closed to the option as far as I can see.

When I arrive home, Bruce is watching a film. He looks tired. I think better of trying to talk about the counselling with him tonight.

I am trying to understand why Caroline doesn't seem to believe me about wanting to end her treatment. Every time stopping comes up, I embrace it. Every time she says she wants to go again, I support her. I don't know what else I can do. Every night lately has been about whether or not we should have another go. I've tried to allow Caro to thoroughly explore how she's feeling. We've ended up being totally focused on her. To add insult, whilst I'm doing my very best to support her, she's confiding in a stranger. What I

want no longer seems to be important; there isn't room for me to explore anything. I don't voice my feelings, so that she has space for hers, but now I seem to be hammered for saying nothing. Yes, I dread the endless conversations about treatment, but I still have them. I just try to be strong, keep the money coming in and support her emotional journey. I don't know what else to do. I feel totally betrayed by her going to see Steve. I don't accept that talking to someone who doesn't know us at all is going to help. We need to have the conversations between ourselves. That's the only way I can see of making joint decisions about our treatment and the impact it's having on our relationship.

A little of what you fancy does you good

Bruce and I spend all weekend getting the spare room ready for our new lodger – we've signed a contract to accommodate foreign students from a local language school. Our first client is staying for two weeks. The spare room needs renovating – the sound engineer very kindly tolerated the baby pink décor, as it meant that he could move in straightaway. We now have five days to strip the walls and floor, remove the worn carpet tiles, sand the floor, re-plaster, and neutralize the colour scheme to make it a little more suitable for a broad range of tastes and cultures.

Doing something completely unrelated to fertility treatment together and being alone in the house due to our other house guest being on holiday makes us feel closer, and we end the weekend by having a little spontaneous hanky panky – which is most surprising and *wonderful.* It's the first time in months that we've made love to be together and for each other – not to make a baby, or to remove or distract us from the emotional pain of what we're going through. I even manage to banish my new taunting voice – *'What's the point of making love, if you can't make a baby?'* It feels so different. I am astonished how far away from those loving feelings we had moved. As we are lying in bed together, I speak without thinking first, but it is well received: 'How about we stop treatment altogether, honey?'

Bruce opens his eyes and turns his head to look at me. 'If that's what you want; if you're sure you've done enough.'

'Have I done enough for you? Will we regret this decision in 10 years', 20 years' time?' I ask him.

'Whatever makes you happy will make me happy too. I keep saying this. I'm being consistent. Why won't you believe me?'

'All right. Don't bite my head off. We'll stop then. No more treatment.'

'Good,' says Bruce, leaning towards me and resting on his elbow. 'Here's to the end of it at last.' He kisses me on the forehead, and then we cuddle each other until we both fall into a relaxed sleep.

Fertility treatment for us has lasted for nearly three years. Now it's just Bruce and me and Barney again. The treatment carries you along; time passes and you just keep going. I feel as if we paid to go on the Magical Kingdom Ride: nice and gentle, goes around lakes, with pretty, soothing music playing all around you, but we turned a corner and ended up in Hell's Teeth House of Horrors, only we didn't notice it happening and we genuinely thought that we'd only paid to enter the Magical Kingdom. The cars gain speed and you believe that you can't get off, but you can.

Broody again

I'm ovulating. Since we decided to stop treatment, I keep seeing pregnant women everywhere. I confess that I did a sneaky ovulation test this morning as I had one stick left in the packet. I had gone to the drawer to throw away the ovulation kit, the pregnancy test kit and the small predictor kit that keeps count of the days of my cycle for me. I stood with them suspended over the rubbish bin, but couldn't quite discard them. I can't cope with the thought that I won't be able to make use of the opportunity to do a cycle this month, even though it's too late to be processed by the clinic. And the thought of having a period in 14 days' time without having tried is tearing me up inside.

I want to try again, but I know it'll mean IVF – nothing else is worthwhile. I'm going to ask Bruce when he comes home this evening.

★ ★ ★

'No, not again honey. I thought you wanted to stop,' he shouts. 'You're *not* injecting yourself with hormones ever again. It made you ill. I don't want you to do it.'

'But can you honestly say that you're really done with this? What if, in the future, we wish we'd tried harder? I'm doing this for us darling. Every time you say you're okay with stopping, somehow I don't believe you. If I'm prepared to have another go, why won't you let me? It might work this time.'

I thought it was over, that we'd stopped. But Caro seems to be saying that as *she* is having a battle with coming to terms with stopping treatment, *I* must be battling with it as well. Over the past week she has started to say that I must be in denial. She doesn't seem to be able to accept that I don't deal with this in the same way as she does; she's assuming that because I don't want to go with her for counselling, I haven't dealt with this at all. I don't think that this is fair.

Out of kilter with each other

Steve is sitting opposite me as usual, in the low, blue, armless chair; to his left are my notes and a clock. He waits for me to respond to his enquiry into how I'm feeling today.

'Our relationship seems to be paying a heavy toll for my decision to have another go. Bruce spent all last night playing computer games instead of coming to bed with me. When I asked him if he still fancied me he said: "If you don't know how special you are, that's your problem." We had a row just before I was due to leave home for this session. He said: "We each try every day to make our relationship better and better." I said: "You don't. You don't." Each time we try to get close, somehow it goes wrong; I can't even define how.'

'Men and women respond to this problem in different ways,' replies Steve. 'Men want their wife or partner to be happy first and foremost. But for women who want a child and are failing to get pregnant, the desire becomes intense and prolonged. They need to understand their feelings. Not being able to have a child, if they want one, seems to affect their identity, femininity and self-esteem.'

'Well if I look at the long-term picture, I've felt ready to be a mum since I was about 26 years old. If you look at the process in those terms, I've been longing to be a mother for *14 years* – no *wonder* I feel frustrated and angry!'

'Quite,' says Steve.

'You know, I want to spend the rest of my life with Bruce. I want our life together to be long and happy.'

'And it will be. Remember, I have complete faith in you. I'm sure that you'll be able to survive this and stay together. You may even discover that you're stronger for the experience as well. You're very courageous and caring and you want to understand the process. It's plain to see how much you love Bruce, so I'm sure you can find a way through this. I'll help as much as I can of course.'

The session comes to a close at the allotted time and I manage to feel a little stronger than when I walked through the door an hour ago. I still don't know how to fix it for us, but I know I've got to keep trying.

A failed attempt at reconciliation

Caro has shared her counselling session with me, but it has just served to make me more annoyed. I don't see how this counselling is helping me at all. If the idea is that we will talk more openly as a result of her sessions, this simply isn't happening. The only opinions I respect, with regard to our relationship, are mine and Caro's, so I don't actually care what his opinion on anything is – it's irrelevant. The best way for us to talk openly is to do what we already do – talk to each other. All this is doing is forcing us further apart, not bringing us closer to resolving anything. It's becoming as if Steve's opinion is more insightful and correct than mine, and if I don't agree, then, in Caro's eyes, I'm wrong, not him. She's talking to loads of other people instead of me as well. It feels like she and I are skirting around the issues. I feel that she's taking everyone else's opinion ahead of mine. But no one knows our situation or journey better than us. And no one else has to live it. So it's up to us, and just us, to tackle it. I feel like they're ganging up on me – I feel like I'm really out in the cold. I have to say something in my defence.

'I've been saying the same thing over and over again. You keep asking me "Do you really want to stop? Is that really what you want?" Each time I tell you "Yes". Really Caro, which part of this aren't you hearing? I'm feeling like it's the counselling splitting us up, more than the actual fertility treatment. Why aren't we talking like we used to?'

'I can't do it, babe,' I cry. 'I'm not capable of understanding or dealing with my feelings without Steve's help. I'm not the same girl you used to know. I don't know who I am any more.'

★ ★ ★

I mention the distance between Bruce and me to Heather in our morning support call, hoping for some advice on my dilemma.

'Well, you're going to have to find a way to create really constructive dialogue,' she says. 'Even, dare I suggest, if that means relationship counselling.'

'Oh my goodness, he'd never agree. He doesn't feel that someone who doesn't know us, or our relationship, is qualified to comment. He says that he doesn't feel that having a third party in the room helps to deepen our knowledge of each other at all. In fact, he's told me that he's beginning to dread Tuesday nights, as he doesn't know what sort of mood he's going to walk into after I've been to counselling on my own. I don't blame him actually; I am a moody cow at the moment and it feels like I'm having a go at him all the time. But you're right, I need to find a way to talk to him without it turning into a row.'

'Well I think you need to consider what you are trying to achieve from the counselling. Is it you that needs the help, or is it your relationship that needs support?'

I book an emergency call with Steve in my lunch hour.

'Coming to counselling on my own is causing problems with Bruce.'

'How can I help?'

'Well, I'm in a lot of emotional pain, but Bruce seems to be just wanting me to pull myself together – he's driving me mad. He says he's dealt with everything, but I don't believe him. Why isn't he in as much pain as me and why doesn't he want to come to counselling with me?'

'Well Caroline, I can't comment on Bruce's process because I'm counselling you. I can talk about what you're going through, and that's what I'm trying to do. All I can tell you is what I've said before – that men and women go through this process in different ways. It could well be true that he's dealt with his diagnosis to the extent that he needs to. You and I need to find a way for you to be able to process your feelings without damaging your relationship. Let's talk about that when we next meet.'

Incoming opportunity

I've started another temporary contract without the stress of job hunting: 12 weeks as an administrator for a PR firm owned by Becky, an ex-colleague who knows we need some support at the moment. This means that I can afford a cycle of IVF, if I can get Bruce to agree. Becky knows all about the treatment and has told me that she will support my decision if I decide to have another try whilst I am working for her.

Finding a way forward

I'm mulling over the ineffective communication situation between Bruce and me. An email from my desk at Becky's feels safe – at least I'll be able to get my feelings out without becoming emotional and causing a fight, or, worse still, totally clamming up. An email might give him the space to reply in his own time and without having to compete with my crying fits.

Subject: My Dilemma

Dear Honey,

I do realize the difficulty my continuing counselling is causing, but here's my dilemma.

We agree that we would like, if possible, a child of our own. I would like this very much, as I would like to go through the whole pregnancy and birth thing and, as you also want, for us to be parents of a child who is at least partly a direct product of our love and genetically connected to me. This may still be possible, but because we have to use donor sperm I have to do this via the clinic. This has meant that my whole life has changed immeasurably, having a profound effect on me, and it's not easy.

When you say that you've 'put down' your diagnosis and let it go, I don't see how this is possible when I still have to go through this process as a direct result of your diagnosis - are we really still going through this together?

I know that I appear to have made a unilateral decision to have another go, but this is based on my feeling that this is what we both want.

I would happily stop putting myself through this, but if I do, we will not have a child of our own - hence, this is why I feel that the 'work' (and it is very hard work) I am doing with the counsellor and on my faith is for both of us. I need to feel that I am not on my own emotionally, but I do.

My dilemma is this: I will stop if you just want it to be over, but that has the inevitable repercussion of us not having children. What do you want to do?

Your Caro xxx

Subject: Re: My Dilemma

OH CARO!

Unfortunately I don't have a solution either – I would like to be a dad and to see you be a mum.

What I find difficult is that this part of the process is forcing a huge distance between us and I don't know how to close it. The process is overshadowing every part of our lives, and until we can get out from under that cloud we stand little chance of getting us back.

Look at us – we are talking about this via email and that's no good. We've always talked about everything together, no matter how challenging. Why are you doing this now?

But anyway, to answer your dilemma honey: every time we talk about going back into the 'programme' my heart sinks, not because I don't want to have a baby, but because it feels like the time we can spend finding us again is getting further away. Talking about doing a cycle seems never-ending, in a way that actually *doing* a cycle doesn't.

So what do I want to do?

I want to get us back!! That is more important to me than anything else. The longer this is going on, the further apart we are getting. Neither of us wants that and neither of us knows how to stop it happening. Any of the solutions we have talked about only seem to be nipping round the edges – except for the fact that we see the need to spend more time together. As we have both said, there has to be enough time spare in our lives for us not to be under pressure – in the 'quick we've got ten minutes, let's enjoy ourselves now' school of things.

The difficulty is that not getting pregnant doesn't feel like it will be a resolution, and therefore it is difficult to imagine how we can put it down and go on to be blissfully happy again.

My solution (which practically I don't know how we make work!!) is that we have to decide soon what we are going to do. If we are going to give it another go – great, let's do it! If we aren't, that also needs to be great, and I don't know how we do that.

I LOVE YOU and I want us to be happy, and you to be happy and me to be happy. I am happy, nay delighted, either to give it another go or to stop treatment altogether, if doing either of those things gets us out of the limbo I feel we are in.

I absolutely know that the counselling is helping you move through the healing process as you need to; I do know that you are working so hard for us by doing it. In the beginning I felt that it really was helping me as well, but as time has gone on, I feel it is helping me and us less, and I feel that my 'process' will continue to have a very large anchor on it until we decide what we are going to do – I want to be half of this decision, but because it is you that actually has to 'do' the cycle, I feel that my voice is not 50% of this duet. I feel that I have no choice but to wait until you decide what you want to do – although that isn't the way I want it to be, and I know it isn't what you want either.

I want us to act as soon as we can – to have a plan, get enthusiastic about it and see it through, just like we are great at doing. That plan also needs to look at a whole load of other stuff, including how and at what you will work, because until that is part of it, we won't be happy either.

It's a very big, very hairy monster with pointy teeth, and we need to find a way to make it a pet that rolls on its back to have its tummy scratched!

Let's talk about this more – well, we will won't we?

All my love,

B

Sorry it's taken so long to reply – that's one-fingered typing for you!

15

'Have you thought about adopting?'

To give Bruce a chance to explore what he really wants, we've arrived at a compromise – I've agreed to wait a while before I do another cycle. I'm not going to put myself through injections this time, but will take Clomid tablets, which the clinic tells me are gentler than the drugs I injected last cycle.

To take the pressure off us emotionally, we've decided to respond to polite enquiries by telling friends, family, clients and colleagues that we've stopped fertility treatment. However, what we didn't anticipate is that nearly all of them ask us whether we are going to adopt. A couple of work colleagues have told Bruce that they are adopted, and Barbara and her husband have now decided to adopt after another failed IVF attempt. Her endometriosis has finally defeated them. I'm really touched by the support we receive as people reveal to us the intimate details of their private struggles. It does help to know that we're not alone.

I still don't feel ready to make a decision about adoption, not whilst I'm still contemplating treatment, but I am making myself examine it as an option in case we're unsuccessful again. Of course, Barney is essentially adopted, and he was more perfect for us than we could ever have imagined. But he's a dog, and it's not the same thing at all. Back to square one.

I may sound out a couple of my friends about adoption. I can't believe how many people we know who have gone down this route: three couples in our immediate social circle and some of Bruce's workmates. Maybe I'm being too insistent about the genetic connection I seem to crave. An old college friend of mine has always maintained that adoption would be her preference; she's never wanted to be pregnant or give birth. When she's ready, she plans to adopt from abroad.

Donor sperm will always fertilize – or so I thought

Another dog owner, called Ronke, with whom I have circuited the park on many previous occasions without really asking about her life in any depth, caught me on a bad day and I told her about our fertility problems. She revealed that she has also had fertility treatment. It's remarkable how *many* of the people I come into contact with each day on a casual basis are affected by this issue, and are prepared to share their experiences with me.

In the course of our two-kilometre stroll with the dogs, we touched on many topics of conversation, both emotionally affecting and also light-hearted, including her hobby of restoring antiques. Our walk ended with an invitation from me to help herself to some specialist furniture wax that we bought in bulk to restore some second-hand furniture. She came round to the house last night and we started talking again about her experiences of fertility treatment in the early 1990s.

She was in her late teens when diagnosed with cancer of the long bones. She beat the disease, but was left with fertility problems as a result of the chemotherapy. She told me that she was prepared to do anything to have a family, so she was given an option to remove and freeze ten of her eggs – five for later fertilization with donor sperm, using the IVF technique, and five for an ICSI procedure with her husband's sperm, which had motility problems. At that time, unfertilized eggs could be frozen but were less stable and often did less well when thawed.

The five eggs put together with her husband's sperm didn't fertilize, but nor did those from the donor. This possibility hadn't occurred to me. I had assumed that top-quality, grade 'A' donor sperm would automatically fertilize if the eggs were also good.

Ronke failed to achieve a pregnancy and eventually decided to give up, and applied to adopt, a process taking just over two years; she and her husband are also registered foster carers. I asked whether her desire to conceive her own child was satisfied, or reduced, by the adoption of her two children, who are toddlers and not biologically related to her or her husband.

'At first,' she confessed, 'my biological urge to be pregnant and to experience birth didn't abate.' She quickly qualified this comment with, 'This had nothing to do with how much I love my adopted children.'

She has since adopted a third child: a baby and full sibling to the older ones. She feels that her family is now complete.

Her comments made me think. But despite her relatively positive experience, rather than encourage me to adopt, they confirmed that my desire for a pregnancy needs to be dealt with before I can consider any of the other options open to us. At least by taking advantage of the clinic counselling service I can hope to explore the feelings of loss I'm experiencing, and perhaps even deal with this strong biological urge to bear a child.

Exploring the nature of raising a family

Two helpful thoughts came to me today.

1. Wanting a baby is not the same as having to continue treatment.
2. Mother Nature is driving this, and my biological clock takes no account of the reality of our circumstances.

I went to chant and have lunch at my Buddhist centre today and bumped into Harry, a long-time friend who works there full time. He suggested that we go for a walk in the grounds and talk after lunch. We have been catching up on our respective news and, having paused to stroke the horses grazing in an adjoining paddock, find ourselves in the Garden of Remembrance. We are sitting side-by-side on a plain wooden bench. I tell Harry that I'm going to stop treatment and do nothing else. He questions my reasons and, like everyone else, is now sounding me out on adoption.

'I don't see the difference between having your own child and adopting someone else's, Caroline. Surely having a child is an altruistic act entirely. Either you want to raise a child and be a mother, or you don't.'

This seems to be the view of most people who aren't faced with our situation. I disagree with Harry, and with them.

'The more Bruce and I are forced to analyse and explore our choices, the more we have come to believe that, excluding accidental pregnancies of course, conceiving a child almost always comes out of a self-interest, cultural–social expectations or, at best, the desire to consolidate an established relationship and create a family unit as an expression of your love for each other. It's only once the child is born that your priorities change – or so my friends tell me – and it becomes a life of altruistic love. My friend Marianne – I don't think you know her?' Harry shakes his head. 'When she gave birth, she says that she had no choice but to respond to an overwhelming love from the moment her daughter was born – a biological imperative I suppose, over which she had no control. That's how it should be; that's how Nature intended it.'

'Maybe you didn't want a child in the first place; maybe it was just social conditioning. Maybe not getting pregnant will be protection for your relationship in the long run.'

'Oh, not you as well! I give up. My friends all tell me that a child changes your life. A baby inevitably becomes the centre of your life: a baby needs you as nothing has ever needed you before. It's easy to make choices about lifestyle faced with dependants and responsibilities – especially if you love them with all your heart and they're your flesh and blood. But we haven't been in that situation. We've had to analyse it all outside of parenthood. If we were able to have a child made from the genes of both of us, conceiving naturally…' *I'm exasperated.* 'Of course we genuinely wanted children. But we *can't have them.*'

Harry puts his arm around my shoulders and instantly apologizes for upsetting me. Amidst my tears I apologize as well. I know that Harry loves children, all children, and is a very popular and willing baby-sitter for many of the families in the surrounding area. He told me quite recently that he is one of the 95 per cent of men with cystic fibrosis who are infertile because they have no vas deferens. Apparently it's a condition called CBAVD, which I guessed could stand for Complete Bloody Absence of Vas Deferens. Harry corrected me, laughing affectionately, as it really stands for **c**ongenital (present from birth, but not necessarily genetic) **b**ilateral (affecting both sides) **a**bsence of the **v**as **d**eferens.

Life expectancy for cystic fibrosis sufferers used to be around 30 years, but science has advanced this. A smaller percentage of women with the condition are also affected because they produce thick cervical mucus, or have menstrual irregularities, so the issue of infertility affects their relationships as well.

Harry's just met the girl he wants to marry, and will soon face a dilemma similar to the one facing Bruce and me. We get up from the bench and begin to make our way back to the main house. His arm is still around my waist as he begins to talk again.

'I suppose I'm lucky really. The first aim I had, being born with cystic fibrosis, was to stave off infection and live as long as possible with the support of my family. I never dreamed that I would get married and entertain the possibility of a family of my own.'

We reach the large, oak double doors leading to the lobby, holding hands now, prior to a parting embrace.

'So you'll have no hesitation in adopting?' I ask.

'No, none whatsoever. Tricia feels the same. If we can have our own child using advanced techniques then great, but if we decide to adopt then... It has the added advantage for us of removing the risk of our child inheriting my condition.'

'I envy your certainty, Harry,' I say, giving him a kiss on the cheek.

'Keep well,' he says, 'and make the decision from your heart. If it's from your heart, it'll be the right decision, not only for you, but also for everyone. Keep being true to yourself. It takes courage, but it'll be worth it.'

I walk away across the sweeping gravel pathway, grabbing tissues from my pocket as I go. I wonder if what Harry says is true for Bruce and me. Perhaps not getting pregnant is protection for our relationship. Would just being together as a couple make us happiest of all? If that is the path for us, then we have to make that tough decision together. Bruce has to know that his infertility makes not a shred of difference to how much I love the bones of him. Harry told me to have courage – that word again.

★ ★ ★

I'm on the computer trying to find support groups. The HFEA provides a link to Infertility Network UK, with an option to join them, and one to More to Life – an organization for the involuntarily childless. I'm not childless yet, so not relevant. But I may as well look up adoption while I'm logged on... It'll be interesting to see how I feel, looking at pictures of babies.

Our lives have focused on trying to have a family for three years now. From talking to Ronke and Barbara, who's going through the process right now, adoption involves close scrutiny by social services over a couple of years. As I suspected, you can't apply to adopt unless you've stopped fertility treatment, which makes total sense to me, mainly because of the emotional and physical energy that it requires. Agencies are aware of all the issues that arise during treatment and need you to be sure that you have resolved them.

Also, I can't imagine being able to combine appointments, drugs, scans, monitoring and work with visits from social services to assess our suitability. Before I dismiss this option entirely, I'll give international sites a look, to see if the process is any quicker.

As the numerous agencies dealing with overseas adoption appear before me in a seemingly endless list, I click on Adopt International, an agency specializing in babies from the Far East and Russia, plus a cutesy-sounding one – lovewithoutboundaries.com. Both display fantastic, joyful photographs of gorgeous-looking, exuberant children. I feel nothing. I have nothing against the children, but that's the trouble: when I imagine them next to my heart, it's just a photograph. Nothing more. This is not moving me one bit. I wish I felt differently, I really do.

More counselling – putting adoption to bed

I've told Steve about my exploration of the adoption websites and about my conversations with friends.

'This is a bit of a leap – we were only considering IVF very recently. What's brought you to this?'

'Well, to be honest I was getting really fed up with people asking me if we'd thought about adopting as a direct response to my saying we were thinking about stopping fertility treatment. I just find myself seething with anger when they've said it to me. It's as if it's going to be a totally new concept to me and that my response to them should be, "Oh no. Thanks. I've never thought of that – stupid of me really, if I want a *baby.*" I still feel that the whole pregnancy/birth/breast-feeding thing is crucial for me and, as we both know from talking to our friends, most children available for adoption are not tiny babies, or even toddlers, so I continue to struggle with the idea. Bruce gets annoyed with me because he says that I won't talk about the raising-a-child part of all this. To him, the pregnancy is just the beginning – not even the beginning, because what he looks forward to is cradling the child in his arms, watching it grow, taking it to the park and playing with it. But in my world, until I get pregnant, none of the fun is possible. I can't imagine it, because I keep falling at the first fence, so to speak. I know many people may feel that it's a limited view, especially those who can have their own child naturally.'

'And Bruce? How does he feel about adopting a child?'

'Bruce wouldn't exactly welcome the continued involvement of social services or birth parents in our lives. But despite that, he's come around to the idea by and large. But he's not pushing me.'

'So it's a bit of a stalemate at the moment. Is talking about this uncomfortable for you? Too soon?'

'No, it's okay. I admit that being asked about whether or not I'm going to adopt makes me lose my temper.' My hands fall into my lap. 'I suppose their comments push my buttons because my resistance to adoption makes me feel ashamed – as if I have no heart, no *true* love for children. They reflect back to me exactly what I'm scared of. Did I ever really want to bring up a child in the first place? Was trying to have a family all about me, not about the child? But in my heart, I know that this simply isn't true. I wanted a baby very much; I would have *loved* our baby. But I wanted *Bruce's* child first and foremost – who wouldn't prefer their partner's genetic child? So any subsequent decision to raise an adopted or donor-conceived baby needs, in my eyes, to be taken very, very carefully. I need to make absolutely sure that I'm not saddling a vulnerable child, who deserves to be loved for exactly who they are, with any baggage we might have because we couldn't conceive together.'

At last! I know how I feel. That feels good and right. I can stop punishing myself for not wanting a baby at any cost. Adoption agencies are very wise in their stipulation that fertility treatment should have ceased before adoption processing is embarked upon. I shouldn't even be expected to consider this option at the moment.

'I think that's very courageous and compassionate. You should be proud of your feelings and rationale,' replies Steve.

I also find the courage to admit to him that it's fear of failure preventing me from trying any fertility treatment at the moment. He and I both notice how animated I become when I talk about re-establishing the things in my life I thought had been lost forever. He makes a really interesting observation.

'So what you seem to be telling me is that everything is beginning to get better, but I sense that "the baby project" – do you mind that phrase?' he checks.

'No, no. It does feel like a project sometimes, the amount of effort I have to put into it.'

'...the baby project is a little island off the coast of your life. From the way in which you're talking, trying to make it work for you, you keep swimming over to the island, but to you, your life and your baby project are separate. I think what you want to do is to bring the baby project into the rest of your life.'

'I understand what you mean, but in my case I think it's the other way about – I'm stuck on an island, isolated from the mainland of society, and I can't get off the island. I know IVF is the next step, as well as being the best value for money option we have. I know I stand a much better chance of success with IVF. Once I have a few weeks' salary in the bank, perhaps I'll feel that I can go ahead with a cycle.'

★ ★ ★

Whilst waiting on the platform for the train taking me into work, I observed a girl in tears by the waiting room. She was hanging on to her boyfriend's waist for support, her face buried in his neck, seemingly wanting him to hold her tight and comfort her. He looked really uncomfortable. His left arm was holding her waist loosely, his other arm absently patting her shoulder blade. He was looking up at the sky, trying not to catch the gaze of passers-by. I felt sorry for him, trying his best but praying for it to be over and for her to be smiling again.

★ ★ ★

I can't get away from fertility issues. At lunch today, I was chatting to a man whose wife is just about to embark on their second ICSI treatment. He's finding it a struggle to know how to support his wife emotionally. I found myself advising him to do the things that Bruce tries to do for me. The trouble is, whatever he does, it sometimes isn't enough, and whilst I know in my head that he can do no more, I sometimes feel that I'll never be on an emotional even keel again.

16

In sickness and in health

Barbara reminded me that IVF is not going to be £3000, but more like £5000 once we've bought all the drugs. I managed to encourage myself by thinking about egg sharing as an option: maybe I can get a cycle paid for by offering to egg share. The donor keeps some of her eggs for herself and donates some to a recipient, who covers the cost of the donor's treatment, so both women benefit. Think how much good could come of my doing IVF. That would be amazing – all that life, all those opportunities.

But how would I cope with a situation where perhaps the recipient became pregnant but my treatment failed? I'd know that strangers – the other side of using donor sperm, but worse – were parenting a child of mine. I'll have to think about that.

★ ★ ★

The head cold I developed at the end of the last cycle has now turned into a full-blown chest infection and I'm off work. It's embarrassing, having gone in to help my friend, and I know just what a mess I've left her in, but I can't get out of bed. I have a high temperature and spend most of the night wheezing and coughing. I hope it passes quickly so that I can get back to work as soon as possible.

I've had to miss a couple of counselling sessions because of this virus, but last week I told Steve that he was the only one who had given me confidence, made me feel that I can love myself, warts and all. To cope with fertility treatment, you need good self-esteem and enormous support, confidence, strength and courage. Steve told me that he has never doubted that I will get through this. I asked him about egg sharing as a way to afford a cycle of IVF, but I'm too old: they only take eggs from women between the ages of 21 and 35. So that's that.

I did go and speak to my consultant about the drugs I'd need to take for IVF, and the costs. I do tend to have adverse reactions to drugs and that isn't ideal. I wish they'd given a thought at the clinic to the fact that I am sensitive – drugs and food-wise – regarding my general health; they could have perhaps predicted that I would have a harder time of it with these drugs.

I'm not happy to spend more than two months' wages on one cycle of treatment, nor do I want to rely on credit cards with no way to repay the debt. I am very happy to pursue the less expensive, 'hundreds' of pounds, treatments, but £5000 makes me feel as if I'm gambling all my money on one spin of the roulette wheel – something I just wouldn't do. I think that's why I don't want to do it; it's not the discomfort or inconvenience, it's simply money we don't have.

Bruce is finding my ill health difficult. He hates to see me poorly. I'm determined to get well quickly; I want to be back at work and firing on all cylinders again. I want to be well enough for another cycle as well – one more with Clomid tablets this time perhaps, then I'll stop. I promise myself I'll stop.

Caro is definitely driving this. She's still going to counselling, which I still struggle with even though she says that it's helping her, so I don't want to say anything. But why is she confiding in someone who doesn't know me, a man I've only met a handful of times and who doesn't know anything about our dynamic as a couple? He only hears one side of it, from Caro. It seems to be dividing us more and more these days.

★ ★ ★

Three weeks on and I'm still off sick. I tried to go back to work yesterday, but had to be sent home at lunchtime, vomiting. My periods have also become more and more painful of late. I'm hardly bleeding, but I'm in a great deal of pain and have cramping. I'm still planning the next cycle and have received the Clomid tablets in the mail, but it isn't looking good.

My neighbour has brought me a pile of trashy magazines and a newspaper. I'm dismayed by the amount of successful fertility treatment that we're bombarded with in the media – it increases my sense of isolation and failure, or fans the fire that says that it is our inalienable right to have a child.

Looking through just this lot and watching the news on television, I'm reading that the Countess of Wessex, who had an ectopic pregnancy, has now had a daughter – from the first attempt at IVF; iconic Madonna had a baby, Rocco, when she was 44 years old; Cherie Blair had a baby at 45 and was lucky enough to conceive naturally; Annabel Heseltine had twins through IVF; and the comedian Vic Reeves and his wife have twins after one cycle of IVF. It appears to me, in my present barren state, that these women are all featured in the newspapers one after another, glowing out at me from voluptuous, full-colour glossy pages. Even the television programmes that hint at what a struggle the process can become still seem to shove a happy ending in your face. I watched something recently showing a woman going through the trials of IVF, but in the final few minutes of voice over, the narrator informed me that eventually she got pregnant *naturally*. Aaah, *how marvellous.*

I'm genuinely thrilled for each of these women and their partners, but being constantly bombarded with success stories is upsetting and causes me to focus on my own failure. I wade my way through treatment, failing, trying again, failing again and then running out of money. The reality does not match the current media portrayal. Only 20 per cent succeed in having a baby through assisted conception. Friends urge me to 'keep focused' on what I'm doing, but that is really hard when it's not even going to be Bruce's baby.

Do I just want children because most of my social circle appears to be geared around family? Is it that I'm scared of becoming a social pariah? Does my desperation mean that I *want* a baby for the right reasons, or *not*? What are the 'right' reasons anyway? I've never felt *desperate* for a baby until I couldn't have my own, so does that mean I'd make a bad mother? I'd *adore* my own baby, but if I don't have one, how will that make me feel? Nature can't take its natural course in our case. We remain at our 'default' position: we take no action and nothing happens.

Infertility is a formidable adversary. You can't see it, or feel it. Two women receiving the same treatment can achieve different results. It appears so arbitrary.

Steve says that setting parameters is important, but that I also have to allow myself to go beyond them. I said that I would do two cycles when I started this section of infertility treatment. I think I'm happy to have one more go with Clomid next month, if I'm well enough, then one IVF treatment after that if it doesn't work. If my next two attempts don't work, then I'd like to explore what else our marriage could be about instead of being parents. The only reason I'm carrying on at this point is because of my age – time is not on our side. I'm running out of time, all the time.

Bruce has always said that his diagnosis was final; there is nothing that can be done for azoospermic men. For me, it's not so easy to know when to stop, because there is always more that science can offer in the way of treatment. But all this is money and time and emotional stress.

★ ★ ★

Bruce seems really concerned about me now. He's just come home from work and is sitting on the edge of the bed stroking my hair. I ask him what he's witnessed about me during the past nearly three years.

He replies without hesitation, 'I've just seen you being destroyed. I want you back.'

'I want me back as well, but I'm so lost I don't know how to do that. I've seen you working harder and harder just to keep our heads above water, and we're not having fun any more. You're exhausted and dispirited as well. I can see that.'

★ ★ ★

I'm well enough to attend counselling again. I'm sitting with Steve in his office, reflecting on my next course of action. Picking up on our previous discussions about IVF, he would like to know my current thoughts. I'm still undecided.

'Okay, so I *was* scared of IVF,' I tell him, 'and that's no longer true, but it still doesn't seem like something that I want to do. I'll have to see how I feel after I've done a cycle using the Clomid tablets, but my priority is to get fit and healthy again and get a good job that I love. That doesn't outlaw having IVF later on. I don't know. I get very confused.'

Steve suggests a way to unravel my thoughts might be to attend a Mind/Body programme. It's already very successful in the States and is now being pioneered by my clinic.

'It was started by an American doctor called Alice Domar. I believe she's coming to run a weekend course here quite soon.'

'How would it help?' I ask.

'It will help with the negative thoughts endlessly looping in your head. If you're in a group of women who all "get it" then, suddenly, what you're going through is normalised. If you're feeling a bit lost...?' He looks at me questioningly, and I nod in recognition of my inability to sort out my thoughts. 'If you've lost your way forward, whatever that turns out to be,' he continues, 'it can help you find *your* way through the process. If you do decide on another cycle, pregnancy rates are better in Domar groups than in control groups who don't use stress management, relaxation or other mind–body techniques.'

'And if I decide to stop treatment?' I ask.

'Well, the focus isn't actually pregnancy at all – it's about getting your life back.' He hands me a leaflet out of his briefcase.

> Mind/Body techniques aren't a magic wand that will make you pregnant. But they are an excellent, effective way to help you take back control of your life, cope with your infertility in a much more positive way and prepare yourself to make choices that will contribute to your happiness and good health for the rest of your life.

- Session 1: Introductions, relationship between stress and infertility, side effects and consequences of stress and infertility, assignment of buddy.
- Session 2: Relaxation exercises, learning effective communication.
- Session 3: The art of self-nurturance and learning to take care of yourself.
- Session 4: The impact of lifestyle, behaviour and nutrition.
- Session 5: The pros and cons of exercise, introduction to Hatha yoga.
- Session 6: Introduction to stress management, session one of cognitive restructuring.
- Session 7: Day spent with partners, yoga, reducing stress with humour, life road map, paired listening exercise.
- Session 8: Partners attend support group for men, session two of cognitive restructuring.

- Session 9: Emotional expression, coping with, and effectively expressing, anger.
- Session 10: Assertiveness training, goal setting, summary and review.

(Alice D. Domar PhD and A. Lesch Kelly, *Conquering Infertility*, 2002)

'Sounds good. I do yoga already, as well as my chanting. I like the fact that Bruce could be involved without having to attend counselling as well. How much does it cost? It all comes down to what we can afford at the moment.'

'Well, yes, there would be a cost, but you can ask for more information at reception.'

I thank Steve for the suggestion. Other people have recommended acupuncture or homeopathy. I'd love to try complementary therapies, regular massage, anything to help. I'll definitely give these forms of support more thought. If I can get myself to a better place mentally and physically, it might be money well spent.

My health gets worse

I've found that I have not been able to maintain good health very well whilst having this treatment. I'm fairly robust, I've built a successful career in a competitive field, but this desire for a baby has made a take-over bid for my body. I came home from work early today *again*. I'm so ashamed at having to take more time off. I really am leaving Becky in a mess. But I can't help it. On top of my bad chest, a ghastly period started today – I am cramping so much I can't stand up straight, which isn't normal for me. My periods are usually a two-day bleed with a craving for starchy or sweet food a couple of days before that. But now I'm in so much pain that I can't even contemplate calling the clinic to register for a new cycle. I'm at a loss to know what to do, other than make an appointment with my GP to find out what's wrong. I feel such a failure. Maybe my ill health is psychosomatic because I know deep down that I shouldn't have children, but I am refusing to let it go.

Oh no, there I go again, analysing everything to death. But it's so hard not to. What do I listen to? My instinct. This is so difficult; I feel like I am going into another grieving period; I mourn each time I bleed in any case, but this month it's worse because I'm skipping a cycle. The doctors keep saying that we should have another go before I'm 40. We can't; we don't have the money and I don't have good health. I believed I could fix this situation, but I don't seem to be able to. If only we felt we could stop. Have I the courage to stop? Or did I believe that my happy ending could only come about with a pregnancy and a baby?

Seeing the GP – bed rest and TLC

I'm just back from the doctor's, where I discovered that my prolonged illness is just a virus, albeit a persistent virus. She is sending me for a chest X-ray as a precaution and referring me to a gynaecologist to find out what's causing my bad periods. I've asked to see Mr Parkes as I trust him and he knows my medical history. All these extra tests and appointments mean I have to forego the chance to do a cycle this month. Not again, just when I'd psyched myself up for it. I can't bear much more disappointment.

★ ★ ★

I walked up to the hospital X-ray department today. Pinned to the door at the entrance was a poster depicting a cartoon baby looking slightly panicked inside a simple diagram of a womb. The message said, 'Please tell them I'm here!' *Chance would be a fine thing*, I thought. For a moment I was tempted to tell the radiographer I was pregnant, just to see how she would react, how it would feel to have people around you think you're having a baby. Maybe it was also to help me feel that everything had gone according to plan instead of failing again and again. I didn't lie of course; it was only a flight of fancy.

I'm needed back at work. I want to *be* back at work. I hate being an invalid – or *in-valid*, as one of my friends calls it. I'll go back as soon as I'm able. I need to slow down from now on. The doctor pointed out that I've been through an ordeal these past 18 months. She suggested that the virus may be a consequence of being under stress and getting run down.

A further relapse

I went back to work two days ago, but by 11 o'clock coffee break I was throwing up again. Becky sent me home. I went to bed, but the pains just kept getting worse. By nightfall I was in agony and in the morning caught a cab to the emergency department of our local hospital. I was seen straightaway, put on a drip and given anti-nausea drugs, but they didn't prevent the vomiting. I was diagnosed with gastritis and an infection. Bruce is working really long hours to pay the bulk of the mortgage, so I have to manage at home on my own.

I've had to quit my job, out of a sense of fairness to Becky. Bruce has offered to support both of us financially until I'm fully recovered. He's amazing. Our income will drop by 50 per cent if I give up work completely, but we'll get through this together. I really believe that now. We're both fighting this thing together.

With the gynaecologist

My appointment day with Mr Parkes is upon me. It's lovely to see him again. We meet at the women's hospital in the centre of town.

As I walk into his surgery, he leaps up from behind his desk and shakes my hand warmly, taking it with both of his. I smile and answer his welcome with a heartfelt 'thank you' and an update on our fertility situation.

'You know, if it wasn't for you Mr Parkes, we'd never have known that Bruce had options – despite his diagnosis being so unhelpful.'

'You say that Bruce is azoospermic?' he asks.

'That's right. They suspect that part of his Y chromosome may be missing or damaged, although we didn't have the test. They took 15 biopsies.'

'Youch! He was brave.'

'Yes, very,' I reply.

He lets go of my hand and we take our respective seats on either side of the desk.

I explain about the painful periods I'm experiencing and mention, in passing, about my blocked tube.

'Well, I'll have to look into why you're having problems with your menstruation by doing a laparoscopy. That's a surgical procedure where I insert a camera on the end of a long tube through an incision in your navel to look inside the pelvic cavity.'

Mr Parkes explains how he will expand my uterus and fallopian tubes with a special gas to separate out the various parts that he wants to investigate. He continues, 'If you have a blockage…' He looks at my notes. 'You had an infection seven years ago didn't you?'

I nod. At the time, the reason for the infection was never identified, but it caused me to bleed constantly throughout my monthly cycle.

'You could also have adhesions left inside the tube. Perhaps I can clear those for you.'

'Sounds good,' I reply. 'When I was first referred to you for pre-cancerous cells in my cervix ten years ago, you said that they had most probably been caused by, what was it called...? It sounded a bit like a butterfly...'

'Oh yes, I suppose it does; a French butterfly – the human papilloma virus, or HPV. It's a really common cause,' he confirms.

'Could it be causing my problems with the fertility treatment?'

'Well, there's no hard evidence as yet, but it seems probable that even mild HPV infections may decrease the ability of sperm to penetrate the cervix. HPV can lead to inflammation of that area, perhaps blocking the path. But you said that you've had IUI, which bypasses the cervix. So this is probably not relevant in your case.'

Bearing in mind that I didn't have anaesthetic when I was examined for pre-cancerous cells ten years ago, I ask if he uses anaesthetic for this forthcoming procedure. He laughs in surprise.

'Oh, yes,' he reassures me. 'Of course. It's quite a deep operation.' He opens his desk diary. 'Now, when are you free to come into hospital? You'll probably need to anticipate an overnight stay in case you react to the anaesthetic or have any problems with bleeding from the wound.'

We book the first available date next month and I leave the hospital. This blows my chance for a cycle next month as well, but at least I'll be out of pain and may even discover why I haven't been able to get pregnant yet.

When I told Bruce about the operation and about Mr Parkes' thoughts about my fallopian tubes, he gave us both nicknames – Cedric the Seedless and Beryl the Blocked. We laughed about this for the first time in ages.

A surprise for everyone and a return to good health

Mr Parkes told me that the pain around my genital area is most probably caused by a yeast infection. So that means that since June this year I have had a chest infection, a gut infection and a vaginal infection. I have yet to collect the blood test results from my GP to see why my energy hasn't returned to normal yet. But I don't think I need a doctor to tell me why I'm knackered.

★ ★ ★

I have, this week, been through a gamut of emotions, mostly to do with a fear of not waking up after the anaesthetic. I know I have to find out what is causing this physical pain, and that there is no other way to know whether I have an infection or blockage in one of my tubes, but I am really scared about the procedure. I could leave it alone, couldn't I?

Although it's extreme, in a way it would be better if they woke me up after the op. and said, 'I'm sorry, Mrs Gallup. Your tubes are blocked and can't be unblocked.' Or, 'Yes, I'm afraid it was cancer, and we've had to remove your ovaries and womb.' I've been wishing for the onset of menopause symptoms, or when they open me up to discover something that means I'd have to have a hysterectomy. I'd be devastated, but I'd get over it: the pain would be gone; the decision made. I'm looking for a conclusive diagnosis from the laparoscopy. Bruce's diagnosis was conclusive, mine never has been, which I find difficult to live with. My worst fear is that after all this is done, I *still* won't have a conclusive diagnosis.

Of course, the problem is that I think I *do* know what I want to do – I want to finish mourning for the loss of Bruce's baby and move on. But somehow we can't seem to close the door – the urge to have a child just niggles away at me. It's like having an open wound on which I keep letting a scab form, only to scratch it off again and make it bleed.

Our options are running out. Bruce doesn't want me to have any more fertility treatment – neither do I – and I don't want to adopt. Oh, how I wish it could be that straightforward for me. 'It just is what it is,' as Bruce keeps telling me.

In hospital – one o'clock in the morning

I survived. Operation over, and it's dead of night. I have a very soothing view of the river from the window by my bed. I can't sleep, although I'm exhausted. My mind is working overtime.

I had a bizarre moment just before the procedure. The nurse registering my admittance and taking my medical history insisted on me taking a pregnancy test. I refused, saying that it was 'highly unlikely' that I could be pregnant because we hadn't had intercourse since the start of my last period. Bruce pointed out to me, in a bemused whisper, 'Honey, it's highly unlikely anyway. You can't be pregnant because I have no *sperm*.' It seems that I still haven't come to terms with his diagnosis even now. I keep forgetting this fact – for that is what it is – and secretly hoping for a miracle.

When I told Mr Parkes about the nurse's request, he told me that everyone is asked to do a test these days. Apparently even a 65-year-old woman was asked; she was just flattered!

Follow-up appointment with Mr Parkes

I'm here to have the stitch removed from my belly button and to learn about the results of the operation. Apparently the entrance to my womb was very narrow. Mr Parkes told me that it was so narrow that the painful periods were most likely to have been caused by not enough space for the menstrual blood to escape from my uterus. He looked at my fallopian tubes: there were some adhesions in the right-hand tube, probably from the previous infection, and the small, finger-like fimbriae that 'capture' the follicles when you ovulate had closed over the end. This would have prevented the dye spilling out from the end of the fallopian tube when I had the HSG. He was able to open them out again. So Beryl the Blocked has gone and Caroline in the Clear has returned to fight infertility another day.

I'm so glad it's sorted. I'm grateful to have an end to the pain, if nothing else. If we have fertility treatment again, there's now one less reason for it to fail.

17

'I don't know how to tell you this...'

Throughout this treatment, I have been feeling well supported by Cathy, Marianne and Fiona, who all live locally. They call me on the telephone or come round to see me on a regular basis. Amy has also recently joined our group. She has two teenage children and is a fellow dog owner, so we've been walking in the park together almost every day. I've been around to her house for supper when Bruce has been working late or away from home.

However, for the past six or seven weeks, I've called her to try to meet up, only to be greeted by her answer machine, which seems to be permanently switched on. I really thought that I must have done something to upset her, because she didn't return any of my calls. I couldn't think what I could have done, so I called Cathy, who sounded quite flustered on hearing my voice. She told me that she thought Amy was dealing with a *family issue*, and asked me if she could call me back later.

Still mystified, I am writing at my desk and Barney begins barking his special 'postman bark' and pads off towards the front door. As I open it, sliding him out of the way, I catch Amy scrambling onto her bicycle, closing my garden gate behind her whilst trying to sit on the saddle and push the peddles.

'Hello Amy,' I call, dashing after her. 'Where have you been? Is everything all right? Have I done something...?'

She continues to cycle away, calling back over her shoulder, 'I've put a letter...it's in your box.' And she's gone; disappeared around the corner. *I must have really upset her. What on earth could I have done?*

My heart is thumping as I get the keys for the post-box, which is screwed to the wall in our porch. I lift out a handwritten note: 'To Caroline and Bruce'. It has a little bird and a heart drawn just above each of our names. As I read the letter inside, the mystery evaporates.

Dearest friends,

Please forgive me for not returning your calls. I have agonised about what I should do. I didn't want to hurt you, or to be insensitive, and I worked myself into quite a state trying to think of how to tell you this. In the end, a letter seemed to be the best way. The thing is that, you won't want to hear this, but I'm pregnant – due in February next year. Fiona and Cathy have known for some time, but I know how much you are suffering in trying to have your own baby, so I asked them not to tell you. I couldn't come and see you any more, because I'm beginning to show and I don't know how you feel about having someone in my condition so close to you.

I hope that you'll be able to forgive my clumsiness. I'll understand if you don't want to talk to me for a while, or if you want me to stay away.

All my love to you two brave people,

Amy xxx

(She's drawn more birds and flowers below her name.)

Before I know how I feel, the phone rings. It's Cathy.

'Hi, I was just calling to see if you're all right. Amy said she saw you. I'm sorry I couldn't tell you about her baby, but she swore us to secrecy.'

'I know,' I reply. 'Well, thanks for calling, we'll speak soon. I have to go now…in the middle of something, you know how it is.' *I'm going to cry.*

'Yes, well busy, busy, busy. I'm glad you're all right. I'll let you get on with your day then.' She still sounds awkward as she tails off and hangs up.

Almost immediately the phone rings again. This time it's Fiona, obviously relieved that the secret is out. Apparently she persuaded Amy to tell me and to stop avoiding me. I understand how difficult it must have been for her to keep quiet, but I'm angry.

'First and foremost Fiona, Amy's pregnancy is about the tenth since we've been having treatment,' I say. 'Pregnant women are a fact of life. Why did you all feel that I needed protecting from contact with Amy, when I'm just as likely to be affected by seeing a stranger with a lovely baby-filled belly in the street, in a shop or at the gym? What benefit is it to me, to remove part of my support network by distancing yourselves?' I burst into tears again.

'I'm so sorry, I really am,' says Fiona. 'I can see now that it was the wrong thing to do. I promise that I'll never again let my friendships be compromised. I'll have more courage next time.'

'You needn't have betrayed Amy's confidence you know, you just didn't need to abandon me because she asked you not to tell me about that one particular aspect of her life.'

Fiona feels better, but when I hang up, I can't stop sobbing. I feel let down, as if my friends pity me and have been talking about me behind my back – talking *about* me, not *to* me. It feels like a betrayal and puts a distance between us. I understand why people with children feel sorry for those of us without, but I'd rather they didn't. There are a lot of us about these days.

High-flyer to housewife

I've been at home for three months now, and it's eight months since my last cycle. Bruce is working even harder to keep our heads above water now that we've lost 50 per cent of our income and spent nearly £6000 on treatment. We've re-mortgaged to try to clear some of the debt we've built up.

I've taken over all the domestic chores that we used to share, including the cooking, shopping, cleaning and filing. Whilst chanting today, I became concerned when I realized how little value I put on the endless round of domestic chores, and how little I feel that I am of value when I'm doing them. Is more of the same what I really want for my life? Having a child will only mean Bruce working harder and, with our already difficult financial situation likely to come under even more pressure, that I will be left to raise our child alone for much of the time. Before we knew that I wouldn't be able to conceive naturally, we'd planned that I would continue with my career. Under the circumstances would I be criticized for doing so, my motives misunderstood simply because of a quirk of nature?

I can't wait to get back to work again, but work where? And for how long? Am I looking for a return to my all-consuming, high-flying career, or tide-you-over, part-time, short-term contracts until we have enough money to try again? Is it over for us? Are we done?

This morning, Bruce has arranged a business meeting with another special-effects painter called Eric. Eric has asked for Bruce's help on a big marbling and graining job for a film to be shot on the Isle of Man. I've taken over some of Bruce's business admin. as a way of contributing to our income and to keep my brain occupied. So today I've started to re-organize our filing, catch up with bills and banking and deal with correspondence. I'll be able to stay out of their way in our office, next to the conservatory.

It's noon and the doorbell rings; Barney barks; and Bruce goes to the door. I take Barney back into the office with me. Enter Eric into the conservatory; with a small girl balanced on his hip. My first reaction is *Oh no, he's brought his child with him.* I then give myself a hard time: *Caroline, don't be so mean; he can't help it. Working freelance and having small children is really tough. If you have a baby, this will be part of your reality.*

She is really cute, has a round face, light-brown curly hair frothing in ringlets around her big blue eyes, and is dressed all 'cuddly' in a hand-knitted oatmeal cardigan, olive-green skirt and lace-up 'Holly Hobby' boots.

'This is Lucy,' says Eric.

'Hello Lucy,' I reply without leaving my seat.

I want to return to my work on the computer, but Eric looks slightly panicked about the fact that he has his daughter in tow. I berate myself again: *I should leap up and go over and make a fuss of her shouldn't I? After all, I'm a woman; I should help out with children.* The trouble is I'm not feeling drawn to the situation at all. I hesitate, consider my options, and then decide to let them get on with it. After all, it isn't my child; it was his decision to bring her, and so he has to look after her.

I tap away on the computer; Bruce makes Eric a cup of coffee, and suggests a video for Lucy.

'Great,' says Eric. 'Have you got the Tweenies? She loves the Tweenies. She's even saying "Eeenies!" now.'

In the absence of a state-of-the-art children's video collection, Bruce finds a Disney video for her – 'Lady and the Tramp', left over from when I used to baby-sit for Marianne's now teenage daughter. All goes quiet in Lucy's world, and the meeting begins.

I can't really concentrate on writing or our accounts due to the talk of paint techniques and the sound of Peggy Lee singing 'He's a tramp, but I love him' coming from the sitting room, so I begin to make phone calls and catch up with emails. Then, a terrible smell wafts up my nostrils. I look down at Barney, who is sleeping peacefully in his bed next to me. *Now, that could have been him; he is usually blissfully unaware of his own gaseous outputs, but they usually pass quite quickly. This smell is intensifying.*

I try to ignore it, but can't, so I go out of the office to investigate. Yes, it's definitely Lucy. If we were in a cartoon, a greenish cloud would be hanging around her bottom. What can I say? I have never met her father before, so don't feel I can say anything – he might feel it a damning comment on his parenting ability. I wander back into the office and start to type with one hand, holding my nose with the other. Eventually Eric says, 'Oh Lucy, have you done that nappy thing?'

Thank heavens he's noticed. He's bound to change her now. Oh no! What if he hasn't brought a nappy! I didn't see him encumbered – like all parents – by a bag of equipment when he arrived.

Nothing happens; the meeting continues, the smell gets worse. I consider how I might carry on with my admin elsewhere – but there is no other room where I can work. In a while, discussions between Bruce and Eric mercifully move to nappy-changing facilities. The garden and kitchen are mooted as possibilities.

'Upstairs. Change her in the bathroom,' I cry in desperation, alarmed that this gag-inducing act is about to be carried out under my nose. 'There are nice warm cork tiles up there.'

Eric takes Lucy upstairs. *Thank you Eric! Thank you so much for being a good father.*

Nappy changed, Eric lays Lucy on our sofa with 'Lamby', her soft toy comforter, and a bottle of milk.

'She'll go to sleep now, I'm sure,' he says.

She really is very sweet, and no trouble really.

'Lady and the Tramp' finishes, but Lucy is still not asleep. As a childfree house, we only own out-of-bounds teddy bears – over-hugged, treasured family heirlooms. I'm racking my brain to find something for Lucy, but I can't, and she's started to grizzle and pull at the hem of her father's denim jacket, wrecking his concentration and disrupting the meeting. It's not her fault she's bored, and it isn't her father's fault that he had to bring her, but I know that they'll never be able to get through the agenda at this rate.

However, I can't think of anything to amuse her, so return to my work on the computer hoping that her father or Bruce will think of something. Suddenly there's a CRASH from the sitting room as Lucy has found something to play with – a long-fronded elephant-foot palm whose leaves hang down beyond the edge of the table, just *begging* to be pulled. She has brought down the plant, the pebbles lining the pot and the soil. We all rush towards her. The men begin clearing up, Eric apologizing, whilst I check that no harm has come to Lucy. She is observing the scene giggling, milk bottle dangling by its teat from her mouth, delighted with the increased activity that this has caused. The plant is restored to the pot and placed out of the toddler's reach. Barney is still asleep in his bed. I give up on work and decide that the men need my help. I rewind our one and only video and sit in front of the television, placing Lucy on my lap.

She feels and smells lovely. I can't help stroking her back, and putting my arms around her waist, snuggling into her. Is this what it would be like? This is nice. If she were my daughter...

But if she were my daughter, I'd have to amuse her *all* day, not just for a few unexpected hours. I couldn't do this for *years* on end. I couldn't sit commenting upon the redness of the sun, the blueness of the sky, or watch the Tweenies and the Tellytubbies – it would drive me nuts. All my friends complain of a mushy brain, and this is evidently how it happens. Bruce would still have his work, but after so much effort to have our child, I would probably review my decision to go back to work after a period of maternity leave. I'd feel too guilty, so I would be stuck at home, doing the domestic chores I hate and preparing meal after meal after meal. She *is* really cute though, and our baby would be my own, *our* baby.

Just as I am enjoying my fantasy, Lucy starts to wriggle free from my knee, having seen Eric walking towards us from the conservatory. He thanks me for my take-over on the child-care front.

'She's never like this. Normally wherever we go, she just conks out on the sofa or chair.'

It seems to me that all children I have contact with these days are trying to help me make up my mind about becoming a mum. They've conspired to try to make me see that I wouldn't really like it – I'd be rubbish at it.

As Eric is momentarily amusing his daughter whilst Bruce boils the kettle for tea, I abandon all hope of returning to work and pick up our washing, walking with it into the garden.

Whilst pre-occupied, I don't notice Eric returning to the meeting and Lucy toddling outside to join me. She heads first for the garden lights, and then narrowly misses a dog turd I haven't noticed and cleaned away. She heads next for the compost bin, which has a section at the bottom that can be pulled open for access to the nutrients. I manage to distract her away from each of her targets just before she reaches them. I then take her chubby little hand and return to hanging out washing.

'Here Lucy, come and help me.'

'Sock!' she says triumphantly as she hands me the stated item.

'Good girl!' I'm surprised that she knows the word and spot a potential game.

'Can you hand me another sock?'

She looks at me and promptly falls over backwards into the herbaceous border.

'Get up, darling. Oh dear. Look, here's another sock.' I prevent her crying by waggling another sock in her direction.

'Sock!'

'That's right, sock!' *She's such a sweetie.*

'Sock!'

'Sock!' *This is fun.*

I run out of socks.

'Do you know the word "pants" Lucy?' Evidently she doesn't. 'Why don't you go and find Daddy?' I suggest, turning her in the direction of Eric.

She soon spots her dad, runs towards him pointing, but then quickly trots back to me, having shown me where he is. I take her by the hand, lead her to Eric's chair and then put away the washing basket. But as soon as I turn away, she runs back into the garden to find me and presents me with a sharp screwdriver purloined from Bruce's toolbox, which is lying open on the garden paving slabs.

'Thank you.' I quickly do a safety check, lifting everything out of reach, then rushing to grab her as she heads once again for the dog turd – I haven't yet had time to clear it up. Lucy heads back inside. I follow.

'Listen guys, you're going to have to keep an eye on her, because there are loads of things in the garden she could hurt herself on.'

By 2.30 I've run out of ideas. Thankfully, Eric has to leave to pick up his eldest boy from school. My child-minding stint is over.

'You had to work very hard didn't you darling?' says Bruce, as he comes over to give me a big hug. 'That must have been difficult to cope with, honey. She's a little tinker, isn't she?'

He's smiling as she waves to him from her car seat. I look at the pot plant, tidy and back in place on the low coffee table.

'Peace at last, honey,' I say. But as we watch Eric's car pull away, I'm not sure how much I like the silence any more.

How can we create a past if we aren't making a future?

We're down on the south coast for the wedding of my father-in-law Roger, his second marriage, to Pat. His marriage to Bruce's mum, Alyson, broke up before Bruce and I met.

We're so happy that they've found each other and that they've asked Bruce to be one of their witnesses. For me, it's the first time that I've been aware of the sheer numbers of the extended family: the immediate family number 22, including Pat's grandchildren – a little overwhelming for this only child.

On the way out of the registry office, I notice that Bruce is looking pre-occupied.

'What is it, honey? What's the matter?' I place my arm around his waist and we step aside from the celebrations.

'When I signed the marriage certificate, I saw that my grandfather's name was cited next to my dad's. It said "Sidney Gallup – Master Butcher; Roger Gallup – Engineer". So I signed "Bruce Gallup – Master Painter". Three generations together, on one piece of paper. But that's all there ever will be. It really hit me. Even if we have a donor child, even though he or she will have our surname, this is the end of our bloodline. I know it doesn't really matter, but it catapulted me back to the awful shock of three years ago. Just when I thought I'd dealt with it, it came back and bit me on the bum, if you know what I mean.'

I can't think of anything to say. I feel the same regret, especially as my own family is so small. I hug Bruce and squeeze him tight, kissing him two or three times on the lips to show him how much I still love him. I hope it's enough.

★ ★ ★

Our solicitor called this morning. We arranged to change our wills to take account of our marriage, but now we're discovering one of the other challenges facing us if we remain childless: where do we bequeath our estate and assets, such as they are?

It made me think seriously of a future without children, well a family of our own in any case. I've decided to try my version of 'journaling' – something suggested in Alice Domar's book.

A Letter to Myself 40 Years into the Future

Dear Caroline,

You're probably sitting there in your big, comfy armchair, looking out over the countryside, or seaside, wearing your favourite purple wrap, the earrings Bruce bought you for your eightieth birthday and the pendant he gave you for your golden wedding anniversary last year. I see your faithful old spaniel curled up, snoring, on your lap and the new puppy asleep in his basket. Have you got time for a quick chat and a catch up?

Do you remember that decision I made back in 2004 not to continue with the fertility treatment? It created the life you have now. Was it the right decision? How has it all worked out? Do you regret not having kids? Should I have tried harder?

I've just finished our third cycle of treatment with donor sperm and I don't think it worked again. Now I want to stop trying. We're out of money, I'm out of a job, and I feel a complete failure. How do you feel 40 years on? Maybe I began to make the decision not to have any children at all when I first realized that I couldn't have Bruce's children naturally, and that nothing could be done about his condition. I always imagined my own child – a child fathered by my beloved Bruce. From the moment I met him, I knew he'd make a great dad and I yearned to be the mother of his children. Raising our children together would have been a dream come true – I didn't even imagine that fulfilling that dream would be impossible.

I always wanted to experience what it was like to be pregnant and to feel that special bond of breast-feeding and nurturing my own child. Have you felt as 'dry', 'empty' and 'unwomanly' as I was afraid you might?

Maybe you and Bruce decided to live the next 40 years alone together. I wanted to travel if we couldn't have kids. Did you do that?

How about Betty? I'm so upset about her not being able to be a grandma. Did she ever show any signs of being disappointed? If she was, she probably would not have let you see. Of course, you haven't had the chance to be a grandmother either. Perhaps you have nephews and nieces now.

I suppose because I stopped the treatment, you had to make a choice about whether or not children were going to figure in your life in some way. Did your outlook on life get very serious? Did you distance yourself from friends and relations with children? How long did it hurt to be around pregnant women? I always felt genuine happiness for them, but wished I could have that sort of happiness too. It must have got easier when you reached the menopause, or did you feel that you hadn't fulfilled your purpose as a woman, that all the eggs you had had were gone without ever being used? You do know that I tried my hardest whilst I could, don't you? I overcame my resistance of using donor sperm, and loved Bruce more and more.

I felt humiliated by all those scans, but have you remained in contact with the fertility professionals who helped make it more bearable? I lost a few friends along the way. Who are your friends now? Still the ones who supported me through those hard times? And have you made a difference to the world? Are you living the life of freedom and happiness I wanted to live, whatever happened? Did you bounce back, as I do now, or were you defeated by my inability to have children? Just thinking back to how much has happened to me in the first 40 years of my life, I can't wait to see what you made of the next 40.

With love and hope, Caroline x

★ ★ ★

'Are we sure, I mean really *sure*, that we're done with treatment?' Bruce asks me, having just read the *Letter to Myself.*

'Four months ago, my answer would have been an unequivocal "yes", but since I've had the chance to recover my health and well-being I'm not sure… We still have time. Do we have the money?'

'Well, I've just had news of the sniff of a big commercial from the construction company. Do you want to put that fee towards another go? Can you bear it, do you think?'

'I think it's about doing as much as we can while we can. So yes, I want to try again.'

'Okay.'

'Right. I'll ring the clinic and make an appointment for next week – one final go.'

'Shall we keep it to ourselves this time? What do you think?'

'Yes, good idea. If we don't tell anyone, we won't get the endless well-meaning enquiries, and if it doesn't work, then at least we'll be able to grieve in peace.'

Bruce gives me a kiss on the lips and I respond by saying, 'Here we go then, once more unto the breach my love…'

We give each other a 'high five' and a hug and I pick up the telephone handset.

18

This could be the last time...

Over the past few months whilst I've been at home recovering, I've become 'Superwife'. The energy I formerly reserved for my career has been channelled into learning to cook. I'm finding it quite relaxing: I have to concentrate entirely on the recipe in front of me, someone is telling me what to do and, barring the occasional burnt offering, it always works out well enough to share with Bruce when he comes home. He's enjoying the gastronomic delights in the week and it's put us back in touch with our friends as I create elaborate, but inexpensive, dinner parties, making everything myself. I'm even making extra puddings and taking them round to hard-working neighbours as a surprise gift. It's making me feel good about myself.

I've stopped drinking and I'm exercising like mad to try to be even fitter when we attempt a fourth cycle next month – probably for the last time.

Last cycle, late-night nerves

Bruce hasn't been able to drum up any work for two weeks now. The sniff of a commercial didn't materialize. Previously this wouldn't have been a big headache, but in these hand-to-mouth days it's a bit more of a problem. He's been very quiet all day. Each time I asked him what was wrong, he'd say, 'I'm fine, I'm fine.' Guessing that he is *not* fine, and taking my cue from the cuddles he's been giving me all day, I decide to dig further. He finally confesses.

'I feel that I've been letting you down,' he says.

'But I'm really proud of you,' I reply.

He repeats his concern: 'Are you? Because I feel that I have been letting you down.'

'I don't know how you can think that.'

He's only been out of work for two weeks – it's the first time ever that both of us have been out of a job at the same time. He's been absolutely superb, keeping the money coming in.

'Do you fancy me still then?' he asks.

'What's brought *that* on? Of *course* I still fancy you. I love you to pieces.'

'Last night I had a dream about you going off with another man.'

'You are the only man in the world I want to be with. For me, there is no other man, nor ever could be.'

Bruce changes the subject, apparently embarrassed by my proclamation of love, but, I hope, inwardly reassured.

'I've been thinking. Whilst going through this process we've met people who have had IVF; it's worked for them, they have ended up with kids – very happy. We know people who have tried IVF and it hasn't worked and they've decided to leave it there. We've known people who have tried it without success and have looked at adoption. We've known people who haven't even gone as far as fertility treatment, but have decided not to have kids at all. None of them is wrong. All of them have made the decisions they have for their own reasons and all of them seem to say that they have happy endings. Therefore what we have to do is to choose the happy ending that is right for us.'

'Absolutely,' I agree. 'There are loads of options, but the important common denominator is being happy with the choice you make.'

Bruce cuts me off, nodding his head emphatically: '...the important thing is that you know what the choices are, and that you make the right one for you.'

We wanted to be able to do this 'our' way. And we are.

'Steve says that our process has been about coming to terms with not being able to have our own baby. I don't mean to sound disingenuous, but Cathy has talked to me about the ability to accept the reality of any situation: if you have lost a leg, no amount of wishing and praying is going to make it grow back; you just have to make the best of the one leg you have. We've decided we want one more try. I don't know about you, but I feel that I'm ready for this final cycle. The break from treatment has helped me a great deal.'

If Bruce really wants to be a dad, then this is the way I want to make that happen, but he then has to deal with his fears for me having a successful and safe pregnancy. Also I have to decide whether I am prepared to enter into all the domestic stuff, actively and willingly. My admiration for parents has increased enormously since I've been talking to friends and family about the realities of bringing up children. I do want to be a mum and for Bruce to be a dad.

I defy any couple to be 100 per cent sure that they want to have children before they get pregnant – they end up giving it a go, and conceiving. Most couples, if they can conceive naturally and with relative ease, do not analyse their feelings, motives and capacity to be parents. But we have had to prove our suitability to be parents and plan exactly how a child may fit into our lives, and the process of being assessed has forced us to examine our motives over and over again. We've had no choice but to use donor gametes. How can either of us be sure that we won't reject a child not biologically related to us, despite carrying it for up to 40 weeks? I can't be completely sure that I am making the right decisions, based on the best information we have via the clinic and our friends. All I can do is trust our choices and have faith in my husband and our love for each other. The thing I think that I have squared with myself is that Bruce and I could be happy with or without children. This is something I want for him and for me. Not because I want to fit into a role in society; not because it's easier that way. I'm not doing it for anyone else, just us, me and Bruce.

Falling at the last fence

My appointment at the clinic with Mrs Storry should have been today. I've had to cancel it because we don't have the money to try another cycle – Bruce's most recent client hasn't paid him in time for us to use the money for a cycle. The payment will be through in December, but my ovulation dates coincide with Christmas, so the clinic will be closed. I've made an appointment to see my consultant on the first available date in the New Year.

My period started today, and even after all this time I'm still disappointed. It was late – day 32; I continue to hope that I'm pregnant if it's late. The connection between late periods and pregnancy is so deeply entrenched. This month I seem to feel a mixture of disappointment and relief. I'm jealous of people who can conceive naturally. I actually felt suicidal yesterday, but the thought of a new year helped me to chase the feelings away. I put them down to being pre-menstrual. This process messes with your head so completely. I read somewhere that fertility treatment patients have been proven to become as depressed as patients with HIV or cancer.

New Year – one more try

At last, Cycle Month has arrived. In celebration of the New Year, I have resolved to laugh more and cry less this year. My ratio for laughter:tears was about 20:80 last year; I feel I need to reverse that ratio. Bruce and I were at the best New Year's party we've ever been to last night: just us, a bottle of champagne, a real log fire and as much telly and cuddling as we wanted – no interruptions. There are *some* advantages to not having kids.

I've asked for a new donor, the thought of which is quite exciting. I convinced myself that the French doctor donor and I might not have been compatible. His sperm may also not be available of course. Changing donors actually seems to help me distance myself from the process a little more. This will be the third donor, so it makes the whole thing less personal. It is hard not to attach a person to the sperm, but if I change donor, it's less likely that I will. Perhaps it's better to have just a code, or not be told anything at all – Extreme Blind Dating. In a way, I would almost prefer to know nothing about the donor this time. However, that's unrealistic, as I know that curiosity will get the better of me. It will also be good to have information to give our child on request if the insemination is successful.

I thought that taking a break from doing cycles, plus knowing what to expect, would make it easier to return to. All I can say is that it doesn't seem to. I am as full of trepidation as the last time. In fact, after two failed attempts, and one cancelled cycle, I'm even more depressed about doing it yet again, but I can't seem to give up and be happily childfree yet. My 'outer' circle of friends seem to understand less as time goes on – indeed, I want to say less, keeping clear of their questions and comments, caring and helpful or otherwise. In fact I have mentally moved several friends from the 'inner' to the 'outer' circle as time has passed. Their transition is usually to do with some unguarded comment, lack of understanding, or hurtful action. I know they try to care, and don't realize the impact of the things they say and do, but I feel more vulnerable these days, and less able to cope with daily life as it is. I can't afford to expose myself to those who can't cope with my situation, or don't listen to what I'm saying. I have developed a system of 'three strikes' on being asked how I am.

Them: 'How are you?'

Me: 'I'm fine thank you.'

Them: 'Are you really fine?'

Me: 'Well, it's difficult, but I'm getting through.'

Them: 'How is it with the baby stuff? What are you doing now?'

Only then do people get the truth of the matter. They've had their chance, they could walk away, but if they really want to know and then come back with some crass or flippant comment, well then, they shouldn't have asked. They'll be moved to the 'outer' circle. Thank goodness that my 'inner' circle continues to grow stronger and more supportive.

★ ★ ★

My period's just started and it is clear that another opportunity to defy science by conceiving Bruce's child has not come about. As my rational mind has always known, I will have to pursue my last attempt at treatment with IUI and donor sperm. Each time my cycle goes beyond 28 days without a period, I half convince myself that somehow we have conceived naturally – Bruce's baby. The disappointment is mild, but still there, despite all my logic. I find it amazing that I can still believe that it might be possible for Bruce spontaneously to produce sperm – just one – and that we will defy medical facts and give others hope. But it's not to be. Instead I'm just kidding myself. I just have to switch off that thought, keep it suppressed as deep as I can to get through this. I only just manage to keep it under control because it's the only way to have a child that is mine, I will be Mum, no one else. I can't think of this as in any way agreeable; I just have to hope it works this time, and then I can forget about it.

Cycle four, day 1 – Clomid cycle

I feel ready – well, as ready as I'll ever be. A sort of switch inside my head seems to have flipped, and I feel stronger, more stoic, and able to cope with all the prodding and poking once more. I started taking Clomid today. Taking that first tablet commits me to the month, in my eyes, so I've bought my seat on the roller coaster once more.

I phoned this morning to confirm my appointment. I don't know what made me do it, but it was fortuitous as someone had made my appointment for the wrong day; thankfully they shifted things around and fitted us in.

A nurse talked us through choosing a different donor, then came the dreaded blood tests for HIV, hepatitis B and C, and hormone levels. It took five attempts, two nurses and one doctor to get blood out of this stone. My veins just seem to run for cover at the sight of a needle.

Cycle four, day 5

Went to see an opera tonight, a special treat to take our mind off things. No side effects so far with the Clomid.

Cycle four, day 6

I was offered a useless donor today. We had requested at least 5 foot 10 inches; blue/green eyes; slim build and fair hair with artistic interests if possible. They offered us blue/green eyes; medium complexion; short, stocky build and a revenue specialist. Did they read the form? It's so far away from Bruce. *Obviously* I don't want to seem ungrateful to the guy who has donated, but *really*: put together my short, Rubenesque genes – inherited from my maternal grandmother I've been told – with a similar man, and we won't get a child reflecting Bruce's physique at all. On second thoughts, with our present finances, maybe a child who understands money may be very handy?

Cycle four, day 8

I feel guilty now. Time is getting tight – I'm due to have my surge within the next eight days – but stocks of sperm are even lower than normal due to the anonymity of donors being removed this year. I was shocked to find that only between about 200 and 300 men donate in any year in the whole of the UK anyway. The clinic keeps offering us men well below Bruce's height.

I had to leave my tall, slim husband to wait for the clinic to ring with any positive progress this afternoon, as I have to nip into town on an errand. I have just returned home to get his update.

'The staff at the clinic are trying really hard, but they've had no success so far. They've tried a second sperm bank and are just moving on to a third.'

'I feel that I can't agree to a donor I'm not happy with. This is our child we are talking about and I have to carry it inside my body for nine months. It's too important to compromise. If they can't find the right donor, then I'll have to leave it for this month.'

What if it's worse next month? To have come so far and not be able to find a donor – it's heartbreaking.

Cycle four, day 11 – scan at the clinic

I've got a feeling that this cycle isn't going to work. I'm debating whether or not to cancel it. I was standing at the top of the hill in our park with Barney thinking, 'If it doesn't work this time, I actually can close it and say "Okay, that wasn't to be".' That wasn't how I felt last summer or even this Christmas, but the shift in my feelings is so subtle.

Bruce says that having closure is to do with doing what you can while you can, and that is not to do with age, but with how much time, emotion and money you are prepared to invest.

Cycle four, day 14 – scan three

Bruce phoned in to our local radio station today, which was exploring listeners' views on the use of donor sperm and the removal of donor anonymity.

I rang the radio station mainly because lots of people were being put on air expressing what I thought were stupid opinions based on ignorance. The topic of the show had been steered down the sensationalist road, suggesting that donor sperm would only be used by lesbian couples, to which the callers responding to the phone-in objected. They had no idea whatsoever that this issue affects many different couples, no idea of why heterosexual couples like us might also need to use donor gametes. Then there were the idiots who felt that couples not able to have their own children should be forced to adopt or, even more weirdly, to care for the elderly! I thought: 'I have a lot of knowledge on this subject actually and they are talking utter crap.' I realize that talk shows need to provoke debate, but I've heard the opinionated minority hijack the debate on other occasions and I didn't want that to happen on a subject that I knew something about and that was close to my heart.

They delayed the news to hear his views on how much he wanted to be a father and our rights to have fertility treatment if we wanted, or to stop if we want to. The producer phoned us back after the show and interviewed both of us for the 'Drive Time' show. There goes our secret cycle – the whole of London knows about my insemination now.

One of the good things to come out of my spontaneous broadcast has been the number of text messages from mates and colleagues who heard it. Messages of support and admiration started 'pinging through' virtually immediately. None of the men could quite face phoning me, but they did want to say something to me, which is fantastic. It means a lot.

Cycle four, day 16

I had my surge this morning, so it's less than 24 hours before my planned insemination. The clinic's persistence has finally paid off. After searching the available stock at *three* sperm banks, they've found a tall sperm donor for us – but not a skinny one. We are very grateful to an academic researcher with brown hair, hazel eyes, a *medium* build, but, most importantly, 5 feet 11 inches tall. Hurrah! Thanks to the tall man for donating – whoever you are. The sample is being couriered over to our clinic tomorrow, just in time for my appointment. That was a close call.

Not only has the law change removing anonymity for donors affected the stocks of sperm available, but now the licence allowing the import of sperm from other countries is being removed. I'm told that it's something to do with the discrepancy in payment schemes between countries. This means that we will never again have access to donors like our previous French doctor, and if donor numbers don't increase in general, then waiting lists for both eggs and sperm are going to get worse. All the more reason to hope that this time it'll work for us.

Insemination day

Bruce held my hand, which was very comforting, but the treatment was still quite uncomfortable and definitely nothing to do with romance or intimacy. I was very glad he was there this time.

Day 3 of two-week wait

The embryos will be six to eight cells big by now. I feel like I've taken some sort of an exam. I know that I've prepared well this time: I've been eating healthily; I stopped drinking alcohol in plenty of time; I've been doing yoga for the past six months and have been swimming and cycling as well. I couldn't have been better prepared. Okay, so I've taken and failed this exam three times before, but this time I've done my absolute best and I expect some sort of reward for my efforts. I wish that I didn't have to endure these 14 days of waiting for the results. It's so tough.

Day 8 of two-week wait

If this hasn't worked, if I'm not pregnant, I'll feel so empty once again. I know that I should be trying to stay positive. Cathy and Fiona have been chanting with me this week; I've been trying to visualize my babies and have even given them names, trying to convey in my prayers how much Bruce and I want them to be here. They are named Richard, after Bruce's favourite uncle, and Rosie, my grandmother's middle name, and a name my mother nearly gave to me. If this hasn't worked, I can just imagine some insensitive know-all saying, 'Well, you didn't want children anyway, did you? After all, you're not prepared to adopt or to do IVF, are you?' But I did want children, I really did. *Oh no,* why am I talking about them in the past tense? I *do* want them, I really *do.*

Day 12 of two-week wait

Just two days before I can do a pregnancy test, but I have to admit to myself that I don't believe that I'm pregnant. I have spots typical of my pre-period acne. I have stomach cramps as well.

How can my body have failed me yet again? The follicles were strong; the sperm was good; my womb lining showed up well on all the scans. Our parents even helped us out with the cost of the cycle – so our babies should see that they have grandparents waiting to love them. This waiting is *awful.*

Bruce has been brilliant this cycle, and we've really been re-discovering what it means to us to be together. I ended my counselling sessions with Steve last month, not to please my husband, but because I felt that I had resolved all my unhappiness and resentment about the treatment. Now that I'm not confiding in a third party, Bruce doesn't feel as if he's being shut out of my process. We had a great discussion the other night about our different needs. He told me once again that he only wanted to talk to me about our process, and couldn't understand why I needed to go to Steve.

'We've always been so good at talking about anything and everything in the past,' he said.

'I know,' I replied. 'But I have been so depressed, so desperate and distraught; I don't think you understand what failing all these cycles and being so desperate for us to be parents has done to me. You just wanted me to be happy, *us* to be happy.'

'Yes, that's true. I just wanted us to decide on a course of action and then stick to it. As long as you are happy, I don't mind what we decide to do.'

'But for me,' I continue, 'I think it's different. I *couldn't* work out what I felt, or why, without professional help; I wasn't capable of it. That's why I needed Steve.'

★ ★ ★

We don't have enough money to buy a new car any more, sports or family, but we have decided to book a holiday some time soon, whatever the result. Two of our friends have a house on an idyllic island just off the coast of mainland Greece and they've offered it to us for ten days, free of charge; we just have to pay for the flights. It was there, on our first holiday together, sunbathing on the beach, that we decided to try for a baby that autumn. It holds a lot of happy memories and we can totally relax again.

Day 13 of torture fortnight

This long phase of my life is nearly at an end, whatever the result of tomorrow's pregnancy test. My stomach is in a knot. I feel dreadful. I don't want my period to come, but it feels as if it's going to. The prospect of not being pregnant *again* is unthinkable. All the qualities I've striven to develop in my character – optimism, tenacity, determination, faith – all of them seem to count for nothing in this. Is conception just a lottery, just luck?

If I don't get my dearest wish, will I end up on the periphery of society, marginalized, isolated? In response to polite enquiries about whether I have children, will I spend my life explaining away our situation? Will it hurt every time?

With immaculate timing, Ian's wife Janet calls to tell us she's pregnant. Bruce picks up the call, but then passes the phone over to me.

'Congratulations!' I enthuse. 'When's it due?'

'October. Ian was really nervous about telling you, but I told him not to be silly – you have to know sometime, and I know that you're strong enough to deal with it. Was I right?'

'So, he or she will be a Libran, like Bruce and my mum. At least I won't forget the birthday. Thanks for being brave. I don't mind, really. I'm really thrilled for you. Actually, I can usually guess when friends ring to give me news like this.' I laugh. 'There's a pregnant pause before they say anything.'

I hang up, after saying goodbye and wishing her well – I have another baby to chant for now. I turn to Bruce: 'How are you going to feel when Ian and Janet's baby is born? What if our test tomorrow is negative?'

'Look, honey,' he says resolutely, 'I love you, and always will. Sure, it'll be tough if this hasn't worked, but we didn't decide to have children to plug a gap in our relationship; our relationship is based on our love for each other. If we are lucky enough to have a baby, then we'll love him or her with all our hearts, but if we can't, then we'll love each other all the same.' He takes my hand and pulls me into his arms and a hug. 'We'll get through this. I promise.'

Pregnancy test day

My period is staying away; so far, so good. As I have only taken Clomid this cycle, there was no need for progesterone, therefore no drug-triggered delaying of my bleed. I should be testing this morning, but I can't quite face it. I've decided to wait until Bruce gets home this evening so that we can look at the result together.

I'm beginning to have doubts about whether I can really be as happy as I feel. Whenever I chant these days, my overriding feeling is one of complete happiness, and the yearning for a baby is no longer there. I keep thinking, 'That can't be right though can it? I planned to have children. I'd be a good mother, and I wanted them. How can the desire have disappeared?' Given my suffering over these three years, I would never have thought it possible.

Can we possibly become a couple who can't have kids and yet a couple who are truly happy? One thing I have learned, whatever the outcome of today, is that I love Bruce and he loves me, unconditionally. We must take care never to lose sight of each other again.

* * *

It's getting dark as I hear Bruce's key in the door, and Barney pads through to greet him. Bruce comes through to the conservatory, where I've been waiting, sitting in front of a tumbler containing a white, pregnancy testing stick with the cap still in place. He walks towards me, taking off his coat, leans down, kisses me and says: 'Hi honey. I'll be with you in a minute.'

He tugs off his work boots, rolls a cigarette, and then sits down at the table next to me. As planned, he called me before leaving work, so that I could do the test and have it ready. In the next few seconds, we'll know if we are pregnant.

As we sit staring at the small white stick propped on its end in the tumbler, neither one of us is in a hurry to uncover the two indicator windows. We share a look that makes us realize that whether or not there's a blue line showing, it doesn't matter. We've got us; our love for each other is intact, and nothing else really matters.

Epilogue: Past, present and future

Over two years have passed since my last cycle and negative pregnancy test. I'm 43 years old and we've stopped treatment. Drawing a line under the process was one of the hardest decisions we've ever had to make, and to a certain extent I'm still in a state of flux. To aid my process of coming to terms with being one of the currently almost 80 per cent of couples who do not achieve conception or live birth as the result of fertility treatment, as opposed to one of the 20 per cent who do, I booked a follow-up appointment with my consultant about one month after my final result, which I found very helpful. She outlined the facts in my case: at the age of 41, I had only a 2–5 per cent chance of conceiving, by natural *or* assisted means. Bruce and I decided that we weren't the type of people to gamble on those sorts of odds without the support of unlimited funds. In fact, we're still struggling financially, despite the long gaps and the caution with which we approached our options.

Our priority in the short to medium term has been to stabilize and consolidate – 'to get *us* back', as Bruce puts it. Among the emotional and financial legacies we now live with, there is one that is very obvious to us: we are stronger as a result of deciding that we wanted to work through this experience, commit to staying together, and be happy whatever the outcome of our treatment. I asked Bruce if he wanted to contribute to this epilogue, but he didn't feel the need to do so separately. He feels that despite going through this process in different ways, and whilst acknowledging that there have been times when we have had quite different views and experiences, we have arrived at this stage unified in our opinions and speaking with one voice.

During our four years of struggle, we have re-assessed our expectations and questioned our assumptions. As I learned, with help from my faith and my counsellor, I lost my self-confidence and, to a degree, my sense of femininity and identity. In not becoming a mother, I have been forced to re-build and rediscover who I am, and who I have the potential to become. After all this time, my feelings still run deep, my frustration is still being purged, but now I'm enjoying exploring a life without children of my own.

I often ask myself whether, if someone offered me unlimited funds and a guarantee of a baby as the outcome, I would accept more treatment. I have come to the conclusion that I like to entertain the *idea* of giving it another try, but when it comes to picking up the phone and making that appointment, I can't bring myself to do it. We return to our 'default' position – and that is a feeling I can live with. And of course, there really *are* no guarantees. How could there be?

Bruce and I have not emerged from this experience as anti fertility treatment – far from it. We are grateful for the opportunities afforded to us by science and fertility technology, even though we chose not to explore all the treatments available to us. We were well cared for, and well informed about all that modern science could offer at the time. The clinics helped us to spend what little money we had wisely, and at no point did we feel that funds were being wasted, or that we were being forced into procedures against our wishes. For us, it was a wise decision to take long pauses between treatment cycles for counselling and reflection – time not throwing money at it or blindly stumbling towards a baby at any cost.

Available treatments are increasing in number all the time – pre-implantation genetic diagnosis, sperm creation from stem cells, ovarian reserve testing, to name a few. As far as I can see, if it's available, affordable and safe, it's all good news. We were able to do all that we wanted to do, whilst we had the time, and we have reached the right decision for us. We hope that our journey will raise awareness of this process, provoke debate and empower other couples or singles to pursue treatment until they have a pregnancy or live birth, or decide not to.

Bruce and I were perfect for each other when we met, and we're still perfect for each other. I understand, with hindsight, that I was never comfortable with the notion of donor sperm, or of adoption. I really wish I could have been – it would have been much less painful and we'd probably have gained a wonderful family. Despite our lack of success, we feel that if we *had* conceived using donor sperm, we would not have had any reservations or regrets.

As for our fantasy son, I know that he'll always be in my heart, and through my own daily activities and interactions I endeavour to bring his spirit of fun and laughter to life, in the here and now.

One of the simple joys of stopping treatment is that, day to day, I don't know where I am in my menstrual cycle. The onset of my period is once more a minor irritation in my life, rather than a mark of failure and a cause for disappointment and grief. I have found that I 'wobble', emotionally speaking, from time to time. My advice to women having a 'wobbly day' is to give themselves permission to say 'No' to invitations to baby-naming ceremonies, toddlers' birthday parties or family events. Give yourself permission to grieve.

I know that our decisions mean a future without our own family, but I have found many other ways to give expression to my maternal instinct. I adopted a companion for Barney from Battersea Dogs' Home – a puppy who needed a home, having been abandoned in a sack at just one week old; I have become actively involved in supporting the youth division of my faith organization; and last, but probably most important, Ian and Janet have made us legal guardians to their daughter, a role we cherish and look forward to becoming more involved in during the years to come. Perhaps having a little more spare time by remaining childless will yield another benefit – being able to spend more time with my own mother and Bruce's parents, which, as the years go by, will no doubt become more precious.

It may be hard for others to understand the choices we have had to make as a couple. We've had to decide whether to put up with the hand that Nature has dealt us, or to explore what science can offer and try to find a way around it.

At some point, you have to decide how much is enough for you. Will you continue until you have a baby, or will you stop, re-assess, look inside each other's souls and give each other permission to call it a day? Do as much as you want to, while you have the time. Make the right choice for you. Make it together and make it with love.

Glossary and abbreviations

AIDS Acquired immunodeficiency syndrome.

Andrologist A specialist in men's sexual and reproductive function.

Azoospermia The complete absence of sperm in the ejaculate of a man.

Barium A mixture of barium sulphate and water, opaque to X-rays, which is swallowed to permit radiological examination of the stomach or intestines.

Buddhahood A state of life inherent in all beings, characterized by unlimited courage, boundless wisdom, compassion and life-force. A Buddha perceives the true nature of life and leads others to attain the same enlightenment.

CBAVD Congenital bilateral absence of the vas deferens.

Cervix The narrow passage at the lower end of the uterus (womb), which connects to the vagina.

Chlamydia A sexually transmitted disease, which can cause damage to the female and male reproductive systems resulting in infertility. Chlamydia may remain undetected for long periods of time. Most women do not experience symptoms, but it can be very damaging to the fallopian tubes and cause fertility problems, pelvic infection, ectopic pregnancy and premature births and can be passed to an infant during passage through an infected birth canal.

Chromosome A threadlike structure of DNA and associated proteins that is found in the nucleus of a cell. Chromosomes carry genetic information in the form of genes.

Clomid/Serophene (or clomiphene citrate) The oldest and probably the most widely used fertility drug. It is an ovulation-inducing drug. Taken as a pill, it tells your brain that you are not producing enough oestrogen, which indirectly stimulates your ovaries into producing eggs. It is used for straightforward ovulation failure in women under the age of 40. Possible side effects include hot flushes, mood swings, nausea, breast tenderness, insomnia, increased urination, heavy periods, spot breakouts and weight gain. Some experts think that the risk of ovarian cancer may increase slightly if it is taken for more than a year.

CMV *See* Cytomegalovirus.

Cryolab The storage facility for frozen eggs and sperm.

Cytomegalovirus (CMV) A member of the herpes group of viruses. Most adults and children who catch CMV have no symptoms, although some people may develop a fever, sore throat, fatigue and swollen glands. CMV is of most risk to the unborn children of women who develop it for the first time during pregnancy. About 7–10 per cent of these babies will have symptoms at birth, or will develop disabilities, including mental retardation, small head size, hearing loss and delays in development.

DI *See* Donor insemination.

Donor A person who consents to allow his or her gametes or embryos to be used in the treatment of others or for research purposes. Although donors are the genetic parents of children created using their gametes, if the treatment is provided in a licensed centre in the UK, they are not the legal parents of these children.

Donor insemination (DI) The introduction of sperm into the vagina, cervix or uterus. *See also* Intra-uterine insemination (IUI).

Ectopic pregnancy A condition in which a fertilized egg settles and grows in a location other than the inside of the uterus; 95 per cent of ectopic pregnancies occur in the fallopian tube.

Egg The gamete produced by a woman during her monthly cycle. The egg is also known as an oocyte.

Egg sharing An arrangement whereby a woman seeking IVF treatment undergoes one cycle of treatment during which her eggs are recovered. She then uses a proportion of these eggs in her own treatment and donates the remaining eggs to another woman. The woman donating her eggs receives a reduction in the cost of her treatment.

Embryo A fertilized egg that has the potential to develop into a foetus.

Embryo storage Storage of one or more embryos for future use by freezing (cryopreservation).

Endometriosis A female condition in which endometrial cells, which normally line the uterus, implant around the outside of the uterus and/or ovaries, causing internal bleeding, pain and reduced fertility.

Epididymis A highly convoluted tube, about seven metres long, that connects the testes to the vas deferens. The sperm pass along the tube and are stored in the lower part until ejaculation.

Fallopian tubes The pair of tubes that lead from the ovaries to the uterus (womb). After an egg is released from one of the ovaries, the fallopian tube transports it to the uterus. The tubes are the site of fertilization in natural conception.

Fertilization The penetration of an egg by a sperm and the resulting formation of an embryo. Fertilization occurs naturally in the woman's body (in vivo) but it can also occur in the laboratory (in vitro).

Fimbria A finger-like projection found at the end of a fallopian tube; plural: fimbriae.

Foetal reduction (also known as **selective reduction**) The procedure in which one or more normal foetuses in a multiple pregnancy resulting from assisted conception are destroyed. The procedure may be hazardous to the remaining foetus(es).

Foetus The term used for an embryo after the eighth week of development until birth.

Follicle A small sac in the ovary in which the egg develops.

Follicle-stimulating hormone (FSH) A hormone produced by the anterior pituitary gland that stimulates the ovary to ripen a follicle for ovulation. It is used in assisted conception to stimulate the production of more than one follicle (ovulation induction).

Follicle tracking A series of ultrasound scans that follow the development of a follicle to see if an egg is developing.

FSH *See* Follicle-stimulating hormone.

Gamete The male sperm or female egg; gametes fuse together to form a zygote.

GIFT Gamete intra-fallopian transfer.

Gohonzon Members of Soka Gakkai International (SGI) carry out their daily practice to this visual representation of the life state of Buddhahood inscribed by Nichiren Daishonin. All Gohonzon are based on the Dai Gohonzon, inscribed by Nichiren Daishonin on 12 October 1279.

Gongyo Literally means 'to exert oneself in practice'. Generally speaking, the term refers to the practice of reciting extracts from the Lotus Sutra in front of the Gohonzon.

Gosho The collected teachings of Nichiren Daishonin (1222–1282). The term literally means honourable writings.

hCG *See* Human chorionic gonadotrophin.

Hepatitis B and C Hepatitis B is a virus of the family Hepadnaviridae that affects liver cells. Hepatitis C is not the same type of virus as B, although it also affects the liver; it is a Flaviridae virus, a group also causing yellow fever and dengue.

HFEA Human Fertilisation and Embryology Authority.

HIV *See* Human immunodeficiency virus.

HPV *See* Human papilloma virus.

HSG *See* Hystero-salpingogram.

Human chorionic gonadotrophin (hCG) The pregnancy hormone; a protein hormone usually secreted by the chorionic villi of the placenta. Its presence in the maternal blood or urine indicates pregnancy.

Human immunodeficiency virus (HIV) A retrovirus (i.e. a virus of the family Retroviridae) and the cause of AIDS (**a**cquired **i**mmuno**d**eficiency **s**yndrome). It affects humans when it comes into contact with tissues such as those that line the vagina, anal area, mouth and eyes or a break in the skin.

Human papilloma virus (HPV) More than 100 different HPVs have been characterized. Genital HPV infection is very common, with estimates suggesting that up to 75 per cent of women will become infected. Cervical PAP smear testing is used to detect HPV-induced cellular abnormalities. This allows surgical removal of pre-cancerous cells or lesions.

Hystero-salpingogram (HSG) An X-ray of the fallopian tubes, which involves the passage of dye through the tubes to see if they are obstructed.

ICSI *See* Intra-cytoplasmic sperm injection.

Infertility Inability to conceive.

Intra-cytoplasmic sperm injection (ICSI) A process used in conjunction with IVF whereby a single sperm is directly injected, by a recognized practitioner, into the egg. Donor sperm and/or eggs can be used.

Intra-uterine insemination (IUI) A process whereby sperm are inserted into the womb to coincide with ovulation (when an ovary releases an egg) to increase the chances of conception. This treatment can be used where there is unexplained infertility, if ovulation problems are identified, or if the use of donor sperm is necessary due to male factor infertility.

I N UK Infertility Network UK.

In vitro fertilization (IVF) Literally, 'fertilization in a glass', hence the familiar name of 'test tube baby'. Eggs are removed from the ovaries and fertilized with sperm in a laboratory dish before being placed in the woman's womb. The clinic may recommend IVF if you are an older woman, you have been diagnosed with unexplained infertility, your tubes are blocked or you have been unsuccessful with other techniques such as ovulation induction or IUI.

IUI *See* Intra-uterine insemination.

IVF *See* In-vitro fertilization.

Karma Potentials in the inner, unconscious realm of life created through actions in thought, word and deed in the past and present, which manifest as results in the present and future.

Laparoscopy The examination of the pelvic or other abdominal organs with a fibreoptic telescope inserted surgically below the navel. During laparoscopy, suction can be applied to the needle to recover eggs from follicles in the ovary.

LH *See* Luteinizing hormone.

Luteinizing hormone (LH) A hormone released by the pituitary gland in response to gonadotrophin-releasing hormone (GnRH) production. It is essential for the development of eggs and sperm. In the male, LH stimulates testosterone production. In the female it stimulates progesterone production.

Menstrual cycle A cycle of approximately one month in women during which an egg is released from an ovary, the uterus is prepared to receive the fertilized egg, and blood and tissue are lost via the vagina if a pregnancy does not occur.

Merional One of the ovary-stimulating hormones containing follicle-stimulating hormone (FSH) and/or luteinizing hormone (LH). It is injected into a muscle or under the skin. When the eggs are mature, a single injection of the hormone human chorionic gonadotrophin (hCG) is given to trigger the release of the egg or eggs. Merional is used to stimulate ovulation before treatment cycles, or for women who have polycystic ovary syndrome (PCOS) and whose ovaries are not responding to Clomid. It is also used for infertility caused by failure of the pituitary gland and in some cases for male infertility. Possible side effects include over-stimulation of the ovaries, known as ovarian hyper-stimulation syndrome (OHSS), increased risk of multiple pregnancy when used for ovulation induction, allergic reactions and skin reactions.

Microdeletion The loss of a tiny piece of chromosome.

Nam myoho renge kyo The practice of Nichiren Buddhism in SGI consists of chanting this phrase together with portions of the Lotus Sutra. Through chanting, we reveal the qualities of Buddhahood in our daily lives and activities.

Nichiren Daishonin Shakyamuni, the founder of Buddhism, confirmed in the Lotus Sutra that all people could reveal enlightenment or 'Buddhahood', a life state characterized by courage, wisdom, compassion and energy. The Japanese priest Nichiren Daishonin (1222–1282) took this sutra as the basis of a practical teaching through which people, regardless of social standing, lifestyle or ability, could establish the life state of Buddhahood in the midst of their daily lives and circumstances.

NHS National Health Service.

Oestrogen The female sex hormone produced by the ovary. Levels fluctuate during the menstrual cycle.

OHSS *See* Ovarian hyper-stimulation syndrome.

Oocyte The female gamete (egg).

Ovarian hyper-stimulation syndrome (OHSS) A serious complication following stimulation of the ovaries with gonadotrophin drugs such as Gonadorelin.

Ovary The female reproductive organ in which oocytes are produced from pre-existing germ cells. The ovary also produces hormones.

Ovulation The process whereby the ripest egg sac bursts to release an egg, which starts to travel down the fallopian tube, where it may meet a sperm if sexual intercourse has taken place within the last four days. Eggs live and can be fertilized for 12–24 hours after being released, and sperm can stay alive and active in the body for 12–48 hours, so it isn't necessary to have intercourse at the exact moment of ovulation to become pregnant.

Ovum The female gamete (egg).

Pelvic inflammatory disease (PID) Inflammatory disease of the pelvis, often caused by an infection or sexually transmitted disease.

Percutaneous epididymal sperm aspiration (PESA) A sperm recovery technique, usually done under local anaesthetic. A fine needle is passed through the skin of the scrotum and into the epididymal region of the testes, and sperm are withdrawn using gentle suction. Alternatively, it involves retrieving sperm directly from the coiled tubing outside the testicles in which they are stored (epididymis) using a needle.

PESA *See* Percutaneous epididymal sperm aspiration.

Pituitary gland A gland in the brain that produces many hormones, including follicle-stimulating hormone (FSH) and luteinizing hormone (LH).

Pre-implantation genetic diagnosis (PGD) A procedure done in conjunction with IVF whereby a recognized practitioner removes one or two cells from an embryo so that they can be tested for specific genetic disorders/characteristics before embryo transfer takes place. If you have had several terminations because your baby had a genetic disease or you already have a child with a genetic disease and are at high risk of having another, you might want to consider PGD.

Pre-implantation genetic screening for aneuploidy (PGS) A procedure done in conjunction with IVF whereby a recognized practitioner removes one or two cells from an embryo so that they can be tested to ensure they contain the correct number of chromosomes (known as euploidy) and not more or less than usual (known as aneuploidy). Normal embryos (euploid) will be selected before an embryo transfer takes place.

Progesterone A hormone produced by the ovary and by the corpus luteum after ovulation, which encourages the growth of the lining of the womb in preparation for nurturing a possible embryo. Progesterone drugs, for example Cyclogest, Crinone, Gestone and Progynova, can be taken after the injection of the pregnancy hormone hCG, or on the day embryos are returned to the womb. These drugs are taken as a vaginal suppository, a pill, gel or by injection into the buttock. Possible side effects include nausea, vomiting and swollen breasts.

Prostate gland A gland situated near the bladder in men that secretes an alkali solution upon ejaculation, which makes up a major part of the ejaculate.

Seminiferous tubules Very long and convoluted tubes of minute diameter which make up the bulk of the testicles. Sperm are produced here and go through a series of repeating cycles before they are finally mature and capable of fertilizing an egg.

Sexually transmitted infection (STI) An infection that can develop during any type of sexual exposure, including intercourse (vaginal or anal), oral sex or the sharing of sexual devices. Sexually transmitted diseases are referred to by medical professionals as sexually transmitted infections, as most of them are temporary.

SGI Soka Gakkai International.

Sickle-cell anaemia A type of anaemia inherited from both parents. Sickle haemoglobin oxygen sticks together to form long rods inside the red blood cells, making these cells rigid and sickle-shaped. Normal blood cells can bend and flex easily, but these cells may block blood vessels causing pain and organ damage. *See also* Thalassaemia.

Sonographer A person qualified to carry out and analyse ultrasound scans.

Sperm The gamete (or mature germ cell) produced by the male, usually through ejaculation. Millions of sperm are present in each ejaculate and roughly half of these will carry X chromosomes, the other half carrying Y chromosomes. A single sperm is called a spermatozoon.

Stimulated cycle A treatment cycle in which stimulation drugs are used to produce more eggs than usual in the woman's monthly cycle.

Sub-fertility Problems that make conception difficult, if not highly unlikely, without medical help. This term also applies when pregnancies repeatedly end in miscarriages.

Syphilis A sexually transmitted disease caused by a microscopic organism called a spirochete.

Tay-Sachs disease A fatal genetic condition affecting nerve cells in the brain. Babies born with the condition develop normally initially, but soon fall victim to a series of mental and physical disabilities, including blindness, deafness and an inability to swallow.

TESE *See* Testicular sperm extraction.

Testicular sperm extraction (TESE) A procedure done under local anaesthetic whereby sperm may be removed directly from the testis by taking several small samples of tissue, or by inserting a needle directly in the testis through the skin (testicular sperm aspiration – TESA).

Testis Testicle, or male gonad.

Thalassaemia A group of inherited blood disorders whose common feature is to disturb the production of haemoglobin. Haemoglobin is a red protein responsible for carrying oxygen in the blood of vertebrates. The condition presents itself during the first few months after birth, when difficulties with feeding, fatigue, fevers and intestinal problems can manifest.

Ultrasound High-frequency sound waves used to provide images of tissues, organs and other internal body structures.

Unstimulated cycle A menstrual cycle during which no drugs are given to stimulate egg production. Also known as a natural cycle.

Urologist A physician specializing in conditions affecting the urinary – and genital (reproductive) – system, who may also be a specialist in male infertility.

Uterus The female womb, in which the embryo develops.

Vas deferens A pair of tubes connecting the epididymis to the urethra that transport sperm during ejaculation.

Zygote A cell that is formed as a result of fertilization, and that contains chromosomes and genes from both parents.

Source: *HFEA Guide to Infertility* (2006/7) and 'Commonly used words and phrases' in *Art of Living*, published by SGI-UK.

Useful addresses

ACCESS – Australia's National Infertility Network is a consumer-based, independent, non-profit organization committed to being a national voice promoting the well-being and welfare of infertile people of all ages.

Telephone: +61 (0) 2 9737 0158
Website: www.access.org.au

ACeBabes – offers support on pregnancy following fertility treatment, multiple births, donor conception for donors and recipients, decisions surrounding frozen embryos, trying for siblings, deciding to end treatment, and telling children how they were conceived. It provides a quarterly newsletter, sub-group news sheets, meetings, personal contacts for specific conditions and an interactive website.

Telephone: 0845 838 1593
Website: www.acebabes.co.uk

Adoption UK – provides information, guidance, support and friendship, 24 hours a day, 7 days a week. The community receives more than 2 million hits each month and acts as a lifeline to many of its 7000 registered users.

Helpline: 0844 848 7900
Telephone: 01295 752240
Website: www.adoptionuk.org

The American Fertility Association – offers support, advocacy, research, education and referrals for those dealing with fertility issues.

Website: www.theafa.org

British Acupuncture Council

Telephone: 020 8735 0400
Website: www.acupuncture.org.uk

British Infertility Counselling Association (BICA) – aims to promote high-quality, accessible counselling services for those with fertility problems. It offers information to patients seeking details of counsellors specializing in infertility.

Telephone: 01744 750660
Website: www.bica.net

Cancerbackup – offers practical advice and support for people affected by cancer. Its range of information booklets includes how cancer treatments can affect fertility and the future fertility of teenage patients.

Telephone: 0808 800 1234
Website: www.cancerbackup.org.uk

Daisy Network Premature Menopause Support Group – members can speak to others who have been through egg donation cycles, both successfully and unsuccessfully. It also publishes fact sheets and a quarterly newsletter and has an annual open day.

Website: www.daisynetwork.org.uk

Donor Conception Network (DC Network) – provides contact and support for people who have children conceived, or who plan family creation, using donated gametes through donor insemination (DI) and in-vitro fertilization (IVF). It also provides support for adult offspring of donor conception.

Telephone: 020 8245 4369
Website: www.dcnetwork.org

Donor Conception Support Group of Australia Inc. – helps meet the needs of families with donor children; people considering or currently using donor sperm, egg or embryo programmes; adults conceived by donated gametes; donors past and present; and anyone interested in donor issues. It also has social workers, doctors and clinic staff as members of the support group.

Telephone: + 61 (0) 2 9793 9335
Website: www.members.optushome.com.au/dcsg

Endometriosis SHE Trust (UK) – understands that the far-reaching effects of this condition cascades down to family, friends and employers. The trust offers support and information for girls and women with this enigmatic and debilitating disease.

Telephone: 08707 743665/4
Website: www.shetrust.org.uk

European Society for Human Reproduction and Embryology (ESHRE) – the main aim is to promote interest in, and understanding of, reproductive biology and medicine through facilitating research and subsequent dissemination of research. It aims to influence and inform politicians and policy makers throughout Europe.

Telephone: +32 (0) 2 269 09 69 (Belgium)
Website: www.eshre.com

Fertility Friends – an online membership support network for the exchange of experiences with other men and women coping with fertility treatment.

Website: www.fertilityfriends.co.uk

Fertility New Zealand – a national network for all those who have an interest in, or connection with, fertility problems, from people seeking treatment, to gamete donors and people conceived as a result of assisted human reproductive treatment.

Website: www.fertilitynz.org.nz

Human Fertilisation and Embryology Authority (HFEA) – a primary resource for all people experiencing problems with fertility. The website covers all licensed clinics in the UK and *The HFEA Guide to Infertility* (updated each year) provides useful information and patient experiences.

Telephone: 020 7291 8200
Website: www.hfea.gov.uk

Infertility Network UK (I N UK) – provides practical and emotional support to those experiencing difficulties in conceiving. There is a regional network and local support groups, and the charity also produces fact sheets and other information, including a video. It has a telephone advice line, medical advisers and a website with news, forums and information.

Telephone: 08701 188088
Website: www.infertilitynetworkuk.com

Information Donogene Insemination (IDI) – a donor gamete association operating in Germany.

Website: www.spendersamenkinder.de

Miscarriage Association – provides support and information about pregnancy loss.

Telephone: 01924 200799
Website: www.miscarriageassociation.org.uk

More to Life – a national network providing a support service for people exploring what life without children has to offer – for both those who are involuntarily childless and those for whom fertility treatment is no longer a consideration.

Telephone: 08701 188088
Website: www.infertilitynetworkuk.com

National Endometriosis Society – provides a helpline, local groups and clubs, a newsletter and other publications, workshops and conferences.

Telephone: 0808 808 2227
Website: www.endo.org.uk

National Fostering Network

Telephone: 020 7620 6400
Website: www.fostering.net

National Gamete Donation Trust (NGDT) – founded in 1998 to raise awareness of, and seek ways to alleviate, the shortage of sperm, egg and embryo donors in the UK. The NGDT is a central reference point for donors, recipients and health professionals.

Telephone: 0845 226 9193
Website: www.ngdt.co.uk

Pink Parents UK – offers services and information to lesbian, gay, bisexual and transgendered families, including those still planning a family.

Telephone: 08701 273 274
Website: www.pinkparents.org.uk

Project Group on Assisted Reproduction (PROGAR) – campaigns in two main areas: for the right of people with fertility difficulties to informed choice and quality of care, including counselling; and for the right of people to have access to identifying information about their genetic origin.

Telephone: 0121 622 3911
Website: www.basw.co.uk/progar

RESOLVE: The National Infertility Association – a non-profit organization established in 1974. The mission of RESOLVE is to provide timely, compassionate support and information to people experiencing infertility.

Toll-free helpline: 888 623 0744
Website: www.resolve.org

SGI-UK and Taplow Court – the British centre of the lay society of Nichiren Daishonin's Buddhism, called the Soka Gakkai (Value Creating Society) internationally. Founded in 1975, SGI is taking an active role in world affairs, building bridges through dialogue and cultural exchange.

Telephone: 01628 773163
Website: www.sgi-uk.org or www.sgi.org (International)

The Society of Homeopaths

Telephone: 0845 450 6611
Website: www.homeopathy-soh.org

Surrogacy UK – formed to support and inform anyone with an interest in surrogacy within the UK.

Telephone: 01531 821889
Email: admin@surrogacyuk.org
Website: www.surrogacyuk.org

UK Donorlink – a voluntary information exchange and contact register following donor conception pre-1991.

Telephone: 0113 278 3217
Website: www.ukdonorlink.org.uk

VERITY – the polycystic ovary syndrome support group.

Website: www.verity-pcos.org.uk

The Zita West Clinic – a multi-disciplinary practice that uses evidence-based complementary therapies for fertility and pregnancy.

Telephone: 020 7224 0017
Website: www.zitawest.com

Further reading

Domar, Alice D. and Lesch Kelly, A. (2002) *Conquering Infertility.* New York: Penguin Books.

Donor Conception Support Group of Australia (1993) *Let the Offspring Speak.* New South Wales: The Donor Support Group of Australia.

Frost Vercollone, C., Moss, H. and Moss, R. (1997) *Helping the Stork.* New York: Hungry Minds.

Haynes, J. and Miller, J. (eds) (2003) *Inconceivable Conceptions.* Hove: Brunner-Routledge.

HFEA (2006/7) *HFEA Guide to Infertility.* London: HFEA.

Ikeda, D. (2004) *A Piece of Mirror and Other Essays.* Kuala Lumpur, Malaysia: Soka Gakkai.

Lewis Dake, C. (2002) *Infertility.* Birmingham, AL: New Hope Publishers.

Lorbach, C. (2003) *Experiences of Donor Conception.* London: Jessica Kingsley Publishers.

Patten, B. (1991) *Love Songs.* London: HarperCollins.

Peoples, D. and Rovner Ferguson, H. (1998) *Experiencing Infertility.* New York: Norton.

Schover, L.R. and Thomas, A.J. Jr (2000) *Overcoming Male Infertility.* New York: John Wiley and Sons.

SGI-UK (monthly magazine) *Art of Living.* Maidenhead: SGI.

The Gosho Translation Committee (1999) *The Writings of Nichiren Daishonin.* Tokyo: Soka Gakkai.

Index